PICTORIAL
O
COMMON SK

Macmillan International College Editions (MICE) will bring to university college, professional and school students authoritative books covering the history and cultures of the Third World, and the special aspects of its scientific, medical, technical, social and economic development. The MICE programme contains many distinguished series in a wide range of disciplines, some titles being regionally biased, others being more international. Library editions will usually be published simultaneously with the low cost paperback editions. For full details of the MICE list, please contact the publishers.

Concise Clinical Medicine in the Tropics
Series Editor: Dr U. P. Isichei, Faculty of Medicine, University of Jos, Nigeria.

Related Macmillan Titles
M. W. Service: *A Guide to Medical Entomology*
J. O. Oluwasanmi: *Plastic Surgery in the Tropics*
F. A. Nwako: *A Textbook of Paediatric Surgery in the Tropics*
A. Adetuyibi: *Companion to Clinical Medicine in the Tropics*

PICTORIAL HANDBOOK
OF
COMMON SKIN DISEASES

ANEZI N. OKORO
MB, ChB (Bristol), FRCP (Edin.),
FMCP (Nig.), FWACP

Professor of Medicine, University of Nigeria, Nsukka
Consultant Dermatologist, University of Nigeria
Teaching Hospital, Enugu

M

First published 1981 by
THE MACMILLAN PRESS LTD
London and Basingstoke
Associated companies throughout the world

British Library Cataloguing in Publication Data

Okoro, Anezi N
    Pictorial handbook of common skin diseases.
    1. Skin – Diseases
    I. Title
    616.5   RL71

    ISBN 0–333–28611–1
    ISBN 0–333–28613–8 Pbk

Filmset by Vantage Photosetting Co. Ltd
Southampton and London
Printed in Hong Kong

Contents

For Dr (Mrs) Eseohe Ayodele Anezi-Okoro

Preface

About one-sixth of all cases seen in general hospitals, health centres and other health institutions are skin diseases. The burden of the diagnosis and treatment of these diseases cannot be left to consultant dermatologists alone.

This handbook seeks to present the common skin diseases in a form to encourage busy medical practitioners, nurses, midwives, health visitors, and community health workers who have to cope with the bulk of skin diseases, to recognise, diagnose and treat them. It also seeks to make available to keen students valuable information when teachers are far away or examiners are near.

The primary and secondary lesions in skin diseases are listed and illustrated by line drawings. Descriptions of the common skin diseases are supported by numerous colour and black and white photographs. The predominant lesions in each photograph are pointed out. Simple descriptions of elementary examinations and tests to confirm what the reader recognises or to differentiate between similar clinical pictures are given. This guides the reader when it comes to the ultimate decision on whether to treat or to refer to a consultant.

Descriptions of simple methods of treatment and accompanying advice to the patients will enable the reader to treat most of the patients, help all of them, and save the wider community by health education.

Acknowledgements

The idea of keeping the text simple so that the handbook would be useful to a wide range of health workers both in their student days and in their hospital or field work has been drawn from a wide circle. Dr Clifford D. Evans and Dr Robert P. Warin kept their undergraduate teaching of dermatology in Bristol University simple and informative. Dr George H. V. Clarke taught with masterly simplicity the fundamentals of dermatology and venereology in the tropics when I was his sole audience and assistant in Lagos. Professor Charles D. Calnan in London and Dr G. Grant Peterkin in Edinburgh took dermatology to the heights of the MRCP without sacrificing simplicity and clarity. To these my teachers in this field, and to Professor Robert Milnes Walker, Emeritus Professor of Surgery, University of Bristol, a constant inspiration, I remain grateful.

The idea of keeping the text simple has been sustained over the years by the needs of my students: medical students, nurses and other health workers in various hospitals, clinics and health centres. To them I also owe a debt of gratitude.

To the team of the Medical Illustration Unit, University of Nigeria Teaching Hospital – Mr Arthur J. Brooks, Mr Agwu Oyeoku, Mr Michael Nwamoh and others – I give thanks for the illustrations.

My gratitude also goes to Mr James O. Akagha who typed the manuscript over and over again as it was made more and more simple.

And finally I am indebted to the publishers for their encouragement and advice, and for their patience with tardy communications.

Anezi N. Okoro

1 Functional Anatomy and Physiology of the Skin

The skin, the largest organ of the body, is also the body's protector, its shield against a harsh external environment, and a mirror of some of the body's internal disorders.

It is a living and active organ, made up of various tissues, intimately connected with underlying structures, closely associated with the transport and communications systems of the body, richly endowed with many vital functions.

All functions of the skin serve protective needs including protection against injurious physical, chemical and microbial factors in the external environment; protection against injurious actinic radiation; protection against injurious stimuli; protection against injurious fluctuations in body temperature, and in water and electrolyte balance; protection against injurious antigenic factors; protection against certain vitamin deficiencies; and protection against disorders of the immune system.

Skin diseases result from failure of any of these protective functions of the skin.

The skin makes up about 16 per cent of the body weight. It covers the entire body surface, and its epithelium is continuous with the mucosa of the external orifices of the eyes, nose, mouth, ears, anus and genito-urinary tracts.

The skin is richly supplied with blood vessels, lymphatic vessels and nerves. It is thus in intimate physical and functional contact with the rest of the body.

1.1 Layers of the skin

The skin is made up of three layers (figure 1.1).

The epidermis, a thin, many layered and wholly cellular membrane with no blood vessels, lymphatics, or connective tissue. Its principal cell is the keratinocyte. The epidermis is derived from the embryonic ectoderm, and the epidermal appendages (hair follicles, sebaceous glands, eccrine sweat glands, apocrine glands, and nails) all develop from it.

Alongside the basal cells of the epidermis are melanocytes which

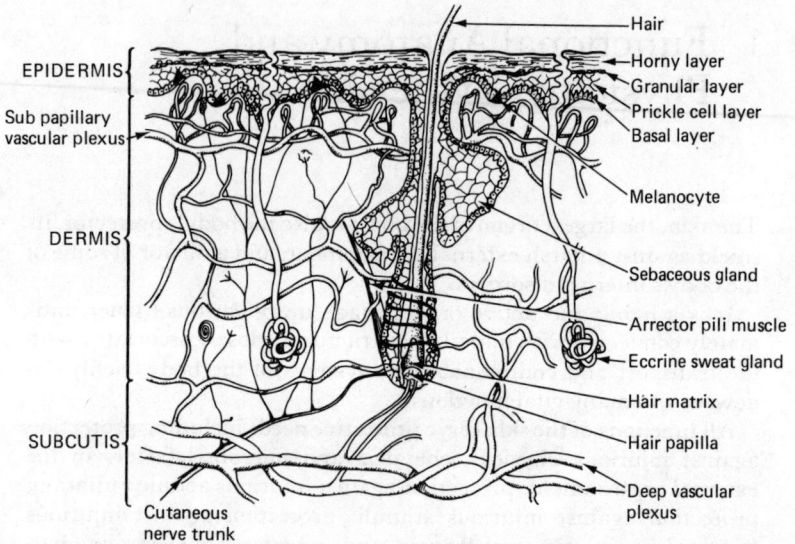

EPIDERMIS

Sub papillary
vascular plexus

DERMIS

SUBCUTIS

Cutaneous
nerve trunk

Hair
Horny layer
Granular layer
Prickle cell layer
Basal layer

Melanocyte

Sebaceous gland

Arrector pili muscle
Eccrine sweat gland
Hair matrix
Hair papilla

Deep vascular
plexus

Figure 1.1   Diagram of the skin.

arise from the embryonic neural crest and migrate through the dermis
and come to rest in the basal layer of the epidermis.

The dermis, a thick dense connective tissue layer consisting of collagen
and elastic fibres, matrix and cells (fibrocytes, histiocytes and masto-
cytes). The matrix and fibres support and protect the cutaneous
blood vessels, lymphatics and nerves as well as the epidermal appendages which dip into the dermis. The dermis is derived from the
embryonic mesoderm.

The subcutaneous tissue which is a thick deeper layer of connective tissue
specialising in the formation of fat and acting as a cushion and
insulation. The principal cell is the lipocyte. The subcutaneous layer
is also derived from the embryonic mesoderm.

1.2   **Variations in skin structure and thickness**

Various regions of the skin show anatomical differences which are
adapted to suit their diverse functions. The scalp, the flexor and
extensor surfaces, the eyelids, the large skin folds, for example, axillae
and groins, and the palms and soles bear various degrees of stress, and
therefore differ in their thickness and in the types and concentrations
of epidermal appendages they contain.

The scalp is rich in hair follicles and sebaceous glands. The scalp epidermis and subcutaneous layers are thick while the dermis is comparatively thin.

The axillae, ear canals, nipples and anogenital regions are rich in apocrine glands and eccrine sweat glands. The dermis is relatively thick.

The palms and soles have an exceedingly thick horny layer and are rich in eccrine sweat glands but lack hair follicles and sebaceous and apocrine glands.

The glabrous skin on the trunk and limbs has thin epidermis and thick dermis and the pilo-sebaceous appendages are not prominent. The extensor surfaces are thicker than the flexor surfaces.

The skin of the eyelids and penile shaft is thin but is rich in apocrine glands.

The skin is criss-crossed by lines, ridges and furrows. Skin eruptions often appear in patterns related to these skin cleavages.

1.3 Functions of the skin

The main function of the skin is to protect the underlying tissues in particular and the whole body in general. Its physiological processes subserve one protective function or the other.

(1) Protection against mechanical, chemical, thermal and radiation trauma.

(2) Protection against microbial invasion. By means of the 'acid mantle' (the thin superficial film made up of horny layer cells and sebum and sweat) microorganisms are usually kept at bay. The skin also protects the body from invasion or damage by microorganisms.

(3) Protection against permeation into the body by noxious chemicals or gases. The horny layer, the granular layer and the prickle layer of the epidermis make the skin impervious to liquids and gases in the external environment.

(4) Protection against excessive heat or cold. The regulation of the body temperature is achieved by control of eccrine sweating, capillary vasodilation or vasoconstriction and heat radiation according to the needs of the body.

(5) The skin is an organ of perception of touch, pain, pressure, heat and cold registered through the vast network of nerves. This perceptive function is protective since appropriate reflex withdrawal or regulation is undertaken following the perception.

(6)   The processes of manufacture of keratin, melanin, hormones and vitamin D are also in their own ways protective. The tough fibrous protein, keratin (in horny layer, hair shaft and nail) is the final product of the keratinisation process of keratinocytes. Other chemical processes include carbohydrate metabolism and lipid synthesis.

The pigment granules (melanin) produced by melanocytes and carried to the keratinocytes protect the skin against actinic radiation and its train of damage ending with cancer of the skin.

Vitamin D manufactured in the skin protects the skeletal system against rickets.

(7)   The various skin secretions: eccrine sweat, apocrine sweat, and sebum have protective functions. Eccrine sweat has already been referred to in (4) above. Apocrine secretions are vestigial supplementary sex secretions useful for the propagation and preservation of the species. Sebum, in addition to contributing to the 'acid mantle', lubricates the hair and skin to give the hair lustre and the skin suppleness.

(8)   The skin acts as a minor salt and water depot and so plays a small role in the control of the milieu interna.

(9)   The skin's inflammatory reactions to irritation or injury ensure prompt protection against extension or spread of the irritation or injury. Injuries to the skin are repaired by epidermal and dermal processes.

(10) The skin's role in antigen-antibody reactions checks deeper penetration of unwelcome antigens.

(11) The skin mirrors emotional stresses such as fear (goose pimples, hair standing on end), shame or embarrassment (blushing, flushing), anxiety (sweating), defeat (coldness). It may also manifest deeper psychological or psychiatric disturbances as psychosomatic skin diseases.

(12) Systemic diseases may have cutaneous manifestations related to the skin outposts of the diseased internal organs, for example, cardiovascular system, nervous system, haemopoietic system and reticulo-endothelial system.

1.4   Lines of defence in the skin

The skin is endowed with a series of lines of defence against injurious, physical, chemical or microbial agents in the external environment.

(1)   The 'acid mantle' (a thin film formed by lipids, free amino acids, sweat and keratin) which protects the epidermis against drying, and inhibits the growth of microorganisms and fungi.

(2)   The prickle layer strengthened by the thickenings of adjacent cell walls and the tonofilaments which along with the granular layer and the horny layer make the epidermis impermeable to water-soluble substances.

(3)   The melanin granules arranged like hoods over the upper poles of the basal layer cells and some prickle layer cells absorb ultraviolet radiation and thus protect the underlying skin against actinic damage.

(4)   The dermo–epidermal junction, an undulating band in which epidermal ridges (rete ridges) project into the dermis. The basal layer cells of the epidermis are attached to the basement membrane of the dermo–epidermal junction (DEJ) by desmosomes, and the basement membrane is supported by a dense network of dermal collagen and elastic fibres. The DEJ therefore ensures a firm union between the dermis and the epidermis.

(5)   The collagen and elastic tissues of the dermis by their resilience assist the dermis in protecting the skin against undue deformity and stretching.

(6)   The dermal granulocytes which chase, attack and phagocytose bacteria and other microorganisms.

(7)   The dermal macrophages which patrol the skin or lie in reserve for battle against invading microorganisms.

(8)   Antibodies or immunoglobulins which are special proteins made by plasma cells. They fight against microbial or antigenic foreign invaders.

(9)   Other components of the immune (defence) system including T and B lymphocytes and complement.

(10)   The overall resistance of the healthy body.

1.5   Causation of skin disease

A breach in the lines of defence, a defect in the immune system, a disorder of the normal physiology, or increased virulence of invading pathogenic microorganisms will lead to disease.

The lines of defence can be breached in the following ways.

(1) Mechanical, chemical or thermal damage to the epidermis and

its 'acid mantle' can pave the way for infection by microorganisms (bacteria, viruses, rickettsiae, fungi) or for infestations by animal parasites.

(2) Disorders of the haemopoietic and reticulo-endothelial systems reduce the skin's cellular defences and combat readiness against infections.

(3) Congenital or acquired immune deficiency impairs the skin's cell mediated and humoral immune responses to microbial and antigenic foreign bodies.

Infections, particularly viral infections, toxaemias and noxious antigens cannot therefore be successfully eliminated, controlled or countered.

(4) Disordered keratinisation, disordered secretory or excretory functions or disordered reaction to the external environment will lead to inflammatory or degenerative or proliferative changes.

(5) Atopic diathesis or other inherited disorders of the skin are often associated with short-lived or chronic or life-long diseases.

(6) Absence of or interference with melanogenesis renders the skin prone to actinic damage and the resultant solar keratosis and skin cancer.

2 'Skin Writing': Primary and Secondary Lesions

Primary and/or secondary skin lesions are usually easily visible. Like Chinese characters, they form pictures and patterns which at first may look bewildering, but are easily grouped into a recognisable 'alphabet'. This 'alphabet' made up of primary and secondary lesions can be quickly mastered. Thereafter, with the characteristic history of the various common skin diseases and the reading of the lesions (single, grouped, patterned, widespread or generalised) a logical analysis will enable a correct diagnosis to be made.

This 'alphabet' consists of macules, papules, nodules, vesicles, bullae, weals, erythema, pustules, exudates, crusts, scabs, scales, excoriations or scratches, fissures or cracks, erosions, ulcers, scars, keloids, cysts, plaques, lichenification, atrophy, hypopigmentation and hyperpigmentation (figure 2.1).

Skin diseases are 'written' on the skin, not in words but in pictures and patterns made up of primary and/or secondary lesions. Primary lesions are the original uncomplicated lesions. Secondary lesions are the results of further development, trauma (for example, scratching), infection or treatment of the primary lesions.

2.1 Primary lesions

Macules: Circumscribed discolorations which are neither raised nor depressed, for example, flat birth marks, vitiligo.
Papules: Small solid raised lumps, for example, acne (pimples), lichen planus.
Nodules: Large solid lumps usually deeply set in the skin, for example, onchocerca nodule, lepromatous leprosy nodule, acne nodule.
Vesicles: Small fluid-containing blisters, for example, herpes simplex, scabies, eczema or dermatitis.
Bullae: Large fluid-containing blisters, for example, bullous impetigo, drug eruption.
Pustules: Small pus-containing swellings. Pustules may develop on their own or from papules, vesicles or bullae.
Wheals: Transient solid swellings looking like orange skin, for example, anti-tetanus serum reaction, urticaria, insect sting.
Erythema: An area of redness or duskiness, for example, drug eruption.

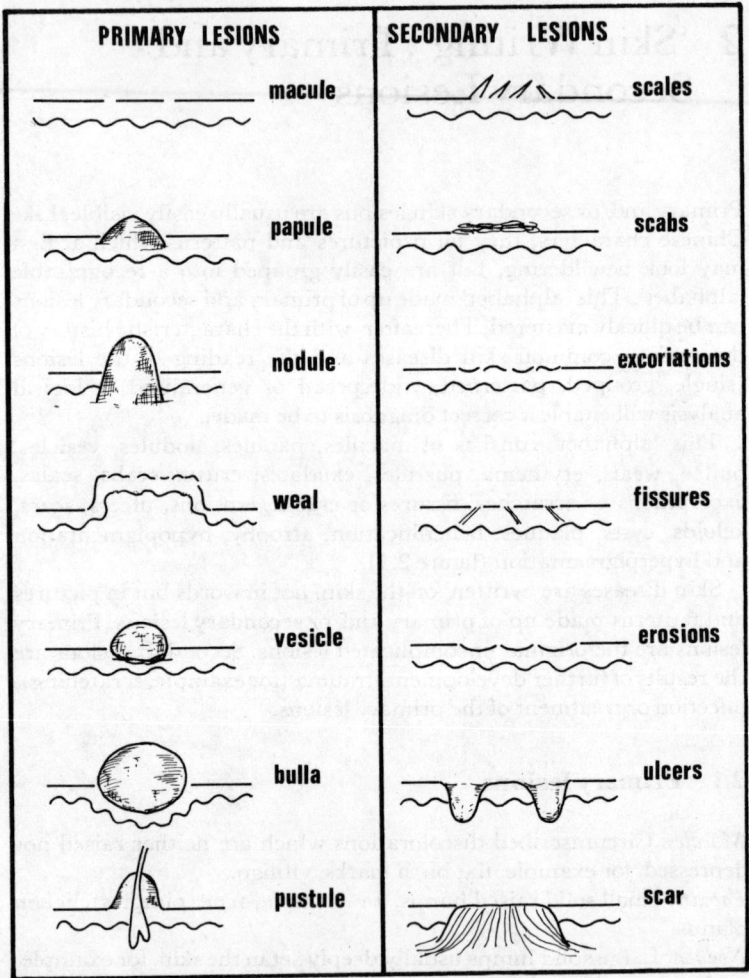

Figure 2.1   Primary and secondary lesions.

2.2   Secondary lesions

Scales: Heaped-up dry horny layer cells, for example, ringworm, eczema, psoriasis.

Scabs: Irregular masses of dried exudate which can be peeled off with difficulty, for example, impetigo, ecthyma.

Crusts: Friable masses of dried exudate which are easily scratched off, for example, broken vesicle, impetigo.

Excoriations (scratches): Irregular marks on the skin showing removal of the epidermis seen in various itchy conditions, for example, scabies.

Fissures (cracks): Linear or irregular breaches of the skin, for example, angular cheilitis, palmar or plantar fissuring.

Erosions: Superficial losses of mucous membrane or epidermis which may heal without scarring, for example, impetigo, herpes simplex.

Ulcers: Deeper losses of mucous membrane or skin which heal with scarring, for example, ecthyma, leg ulcer.

Scars: The end results of healed ulcers. They may be flat or hypertrophic or may form keloids, for example, vaccination scars, surgical scars.

Keloids: Solid swellings on sites of scars, infections or skin tension. Keloids are due to excessive overgrowth of fibrous tissue.

Cysts: Fluid-containing lumps under the skin, for example, sebaceous cyst, acne cyst, onchocerca cyst.

Lichenification: Excessive thickening of the horny layer, for example, filariasis, lichen simplex chronicus.

Hypopigmentation: Decrease in skin pigmentation, for example, leprosy, onchodermatitis, vitiligo.

Hyperpigmentation: Increase in skin pigmentation, for example, lichen planus, neurodermatitis, fixed drug eruption, hypermelanosias.

Atrophy: Loss of thickness or substance of epidermis and/or dermis, for example, chronic discoid lupus erythematosus, insulin injection sites.

Plaque: A raised flat or rough portion of the skin with defined edge, for example, lichen planus, chronic eczema, discoid lupus erythematosus.

3 Common Bacterial Infections

The external environment is teeming with bacteria and other micro-organisms. The skin is the buffer between the body and these microorganisms. It attempts to keep them away from the underlying body tissues and in so doing endures the butt of their attempt to enter the body.

Bacteria get trapped in the extensive net of the skin. Some die off, scorched by the acid mantle of the skin. Some survive and live as harmless commensals. Others become pathogenic either because of their high virulence or because the skin's mechanical or humoral defences break down.

Many bacterial skin infections occur through the hair follicles (the 'Achilles' heel' of the skin). These include folliculitis, sycosis, furunculosis (boils) and carbuncles which are usually localised. Other common bacterial infections occur through small skin injuries or in the intact skin, for example, impetigo and ecthyma which are also localised. These localised skin infections are most commonly caused by staphylococci, and may develop into pyoderma. Gangrene and ulcers are other possible complications of some bacterial infections.

Invasive skin infections usually caused by streptococci present as cellulitis, lymphangitis and lymphadenitis. If unchecked, they may cause a septicaemia.

Common bacterial infections usually respond to antibiotics, the most appropriate being determined by antibiotic sensitivity tests on swabs from the skin lesions, or on the blood culture if there is septicaemia.

3.1 The skin and bacteria

The skin exposed as it is to the external environment is readily invaded by various bacteria which may remain as commensals in the skin creases, folds or hair follicles; or may become pathogenic, enter the skin and produce recognisable infections.

Staphylococci, streptococci, corynebacteria and diphtheroids are among the common resident flora readily isolated from the intact skin.

The healthy intact skin normally keeps these bacteria in check by means of its dryness and the slightly acidic secretions (sweat and sebum).

Factors which favour the establishment of skin infections include trauma (cuts, abrasions, scratches), insect bites, malnutrition, severe illness.

3.2   Impetigo contagiosum (plates 1 and 2)

This is a common contagious superficial skin infection. The face, scalp, hands or other exposed parts which are easily traumatised are the characteristic sites.

The condition, which is commoner in children than in adults, is usually caused by staphylococci and/or streptococci.

Clinical features

Rapidly growing thin-walled vesicles or bullae develop on dusky or erythematous bases, become pustular, rupture and spread to adjacent or distant areas of the skin.

Ruptured vesicles or bullae leave raw surfaces covered with yellowish exudates which dry to form scabs or crusts. When healed, the affected areas are usually hyperpigmented for some time. There is no scarring since healing is by epithelialisation.

Lesions of scabies, eczema or dermatitis or pediculosis may become impetiginised.

In adults, impetigo contagiosum is milder and may present as scabbed or crusted circinate lesions or as crusted dusky or erythematous streaks studded with vesicles.

3.3   Impetigo neonatorum (figures 3.1 and 3.2)

In the new-born, bullous impetigo tends to be commoner and more severe. Large areas of the skin may be covered with thin flaccid bullae in a matter of hours or a day or two.

Impetigo neonatorum may occur in small epidemics in maternity nurseries, premature baby units or children's wards. In neonates, impetigo may carry a high mortality rate unless it is promptly controlled by isolation and treatment.

Death in neonates may result from complications such as septicaemia, gastroenteritis, pneumonia, lung abscesses, metastatic abscesses, osteomyelitis, glomerulonephritis or meningitis.

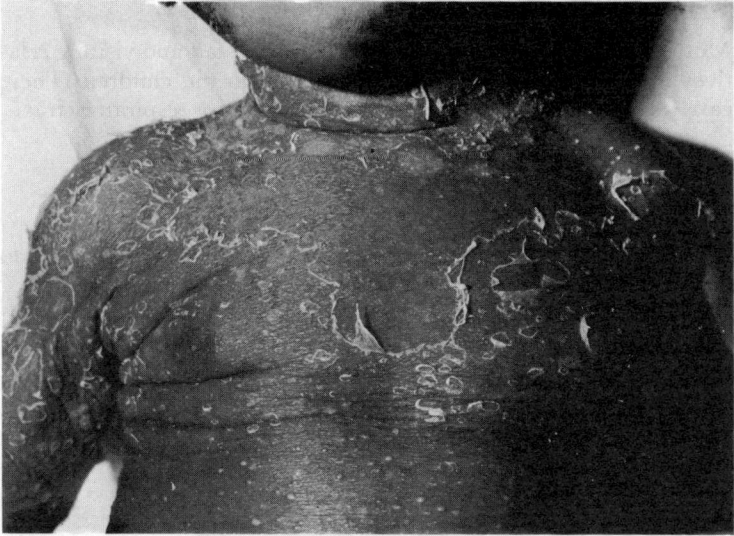

Figure 3.1   Impetigo neonatorum. Broken vesicles and bullae.

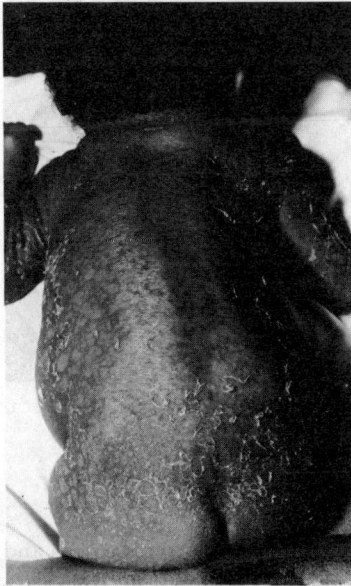

Figure 3.2   Impetigo neonatorum showing extensive exfoliation.

Sources of infection

Mothers, midwives, doctors or other hospital staff and visiting relatives are the frequent carriers of infection to the children. These carriers may harbour bacteria in their skin or upper respiratory tract.

3.4   **Ecthyma** (figure 3.3)

This is a variant of impetigo which tends to ulcerate deeply and to heal with deep irregular scarring.

Predisposing factors include poor hygiene, malnutrition and debilitation in children.

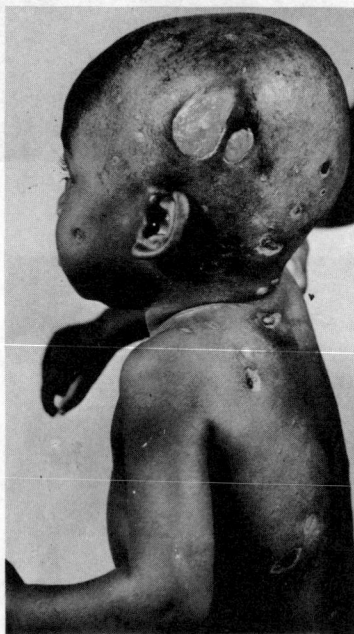

Figure 3.3   Ecthyma, healed with deep punched-out scars.

3.5   **Diagnosis of impetigo**

This is based on the clinical picture, isolation and culture of organisms from lesions and antibiotic sensitivity tests where facilities are available.

3.6 Treatment of impetigo

Topical applications

In mild cases, topical applications will usually suffice after the crusts have been soaked with liquid paraffin and removed with forceps.

(1) Gentian violet (magenta paint) 1 per cent aqueous solution or 0.5 per cent in spirit. Apply b.d.
(2) Antibiotic cream or ointment: neomycin, bacitracin, gentamicin (Genticin) or polymyxin. Apply b.d.

Systemic treatment

In neonates, debilitated children or those with complications, prompt and adequate antibiotic treatment should be given

(1) Procaine penicillin 400,000 units – 1.2 megaunits daily (depending on age and weight) for 5–7 days.
or (2) Crystalline penicillin 1–2 megaunits in divided doses daily.
or (3) Penicillin V tablets or syrup 200,000 units – 500,000 units t.i.d.

In severe cases Ampiclox (ampicillin and cloxacillin) if available should be given orally or by injection. In patients with hypersensitivity to penicillin, tetracycline, erythromycin or other widespectrum antibiotics 125mg–250mg q.i.d. depending on age and weight.

When widespectrum antibiotics are given, multivitamin syrup or tablets should be given to guard against superinfection with *Candida albicans* or other microorganisms.

3.7 Prophylaxis

Accurate history of contact is essential for the control of the spread of impetigo.

Prevention of the spread of impetigo should be by avoiding close contact and the exchange of fomites.

Hospital workers in close contact with neonates should be screened to ensure that they do not harbour pathogenic bacteria in the skin or upper respiratory tracts. Relatives should not be allowed into nurseries.

3.8 Hair follicle infections

The population density of bacteria on the skin is higher in and around the hair follicles than elsewhere on the skin. Bacterial infection of the skin through the hair follicles is common, and the clinical picture of the infection depends on how far down the hair follicles the infection is set up.

Folliculitis Pyogenic infection of the mouths or superficial parts of the hair follicles, presenting as small yellowish pustules at the mouths of the hair follicles.

Sometimes contact with mineral oils, other chemicals or adhesive dressings or plasters may plug the mouths of hair follicles and produce folliculitis.

Folliculitis may also follow shaving especially of the beard area or back of the neck.

Sycosis Recurrent or chronic pyogenic infection of the deeper parts of the hair follicles. This is common in coarse-haired areas of the body, and presents with papules, pustules, nodules, scabs or crusts and surrounding cellulitis, oedema or induration. There may be subsequent development of lymphangitis and regional lymphadenitis.

The four common types of sycosis are

Sycosis barbae – affecting the beard area in men (figure 3.4).
Sycosis nuchae – affecting the back of the neck, around the hair line. This is common in men (figure 3.5).
Sycosis pubis – affecting the pubic region.
Sycosis cruris – usually affecting the anterior and lateral aspects of the lower legs. This is the commonest type and is seen in both sexes (figure 3.6).

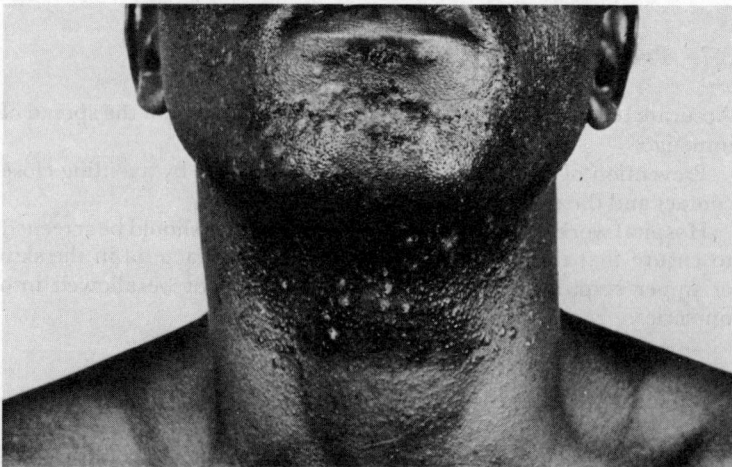

Figure 3.4   Sycosis barbae: pustules and scabs on chin and neck.

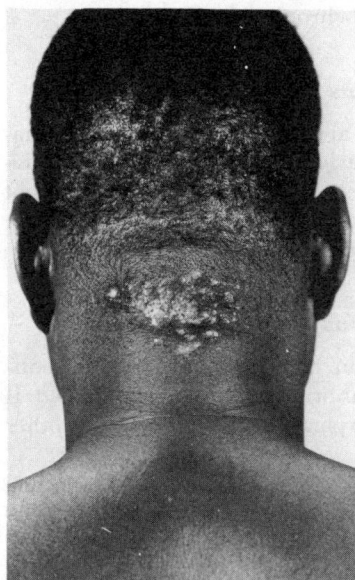

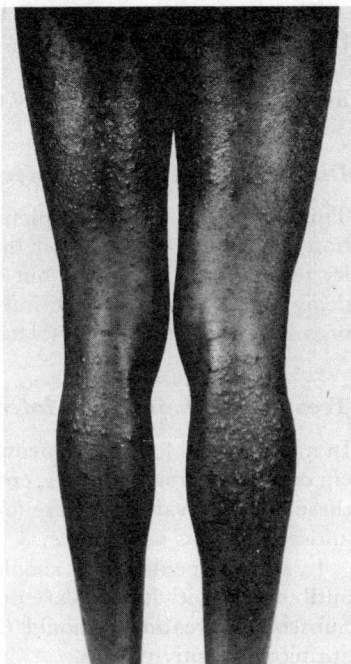

Figure 3.5   *(Left)* Sycosis nuchae: pustules and scabs on back of neck.
Figure 3.6   *(Right)* Sycosis cruris: pustules on lower legs and thighs.

Furunculosis (boils) Infection of the roots of hair follicles may develop into boils.

A boil or furuncle is a roundish or domeshaped tender nodule which usually ends up with central suppuration or necrosis. The common sites are the face and neck, the large folds, buttocks and perineum, and hands.

Predisposing factors include harbouring of staphylococci in the nose, perineum or other sites, debility, malnutrition, obesity, and diabetes mellitus.

Carbuncle This is a deep staphylococcal infection formed by the coalescing of a number of contiguous boils. The overlying skin is dusky, indurated, painful and tender because the inflammation extends beyond the hair follicles to surrounding and underlying connective tissues.

A carbuncle may suppurate and discharge through multiple sinuses or may necrose and slough or ulcerate.

The common sites are the back of the neck, the back, waist, buttocks and thighs.

Predisposing factors include malnutrition, debility, diabetes mellitus, prolonged steroid therapy and chronic skin diseases.

Diagnosis of hair follicle infections

This is based on the clinical picture, and on the microscopic examination and culture of swabs from the various lesions. Antibiotic sensitivity tests should be carried out where possible, but this should not delay the treatment of the infections. *Staphylococcus pyogenes* is the organism most commonly isolated from the lesions.

Treatment of hair follicle infections

In mild cases of folliculitis, neomycin, bacitracin, polymyxin, Genticin or other antibiotic sprays, creams or ointments may be applied. If these are not available or are too expensive, Gentian violet or other antiseptic paints may suffice.

In sycosis, penicillin G should be given in adequate doses while antibiotic sensitivity tests are performed on the isolated organisms. Subsequent treatment should then be based on the results of the antibiotic sensitivity tests.

In furunculosis and carbuncle the lesions, when fluctuant, should be incised and drained or dressed. Penicillin G should be given in adequate doses to be followed if necessary by other antibiotics as determined by the antibiotic sensitivity tests.

Diabetes mellitus or any underlying disease should be treated.

Prophylaxis

Carrier sites such as the nose should be treated with topical antibiotics. The urine should be tested routinely and diabetes mellitus or any underlying disease treated. Malnutrition and anaemia if present should also be treated.

3.9　Cellulitis

This is an acute, subacute, recurrent or chronic inflammation of the skin and subcutaneous tissues usually due to streptococcal infection.

It usually follows a scratch, pin prick, fissure, cut, wound or ulcer or may develop on apparently normal skin.

The affected area may be red or dusky, oedematous or indurated and tender. Streaks of redness or duskiness indicate lymphangitis and the regional lymph nodes may become inflamed, enlarged and tender. There may be associated constitutional upset with fever and malaise. Complications may include septicaemia, focal necrosis and gangrene.

In recurrent or chronic cases, localised lymphoedema may develop.

Diagnosis

This is based on the clinical picture, microscopy and culture of swabs from lesions, blood culture, and antibiotic sensitivity tests.

Treatment

Penicillin G should be given promptly and in adequate doses while antibiotic sensitivity tests are performed to appraise the need for further treatment.

The affected parts should be rested and bed rest may be necessary.

Any underlying systemic disease should be treated.

3.10 Pyoderma

This is a spreading bacterial infection of the skin with a mixed picture of folliculitis, furunculosis, impetigo, cellulitis, granulation and ulceration (figure 3.7). The scalp, face, hairy regions, hands and feet are the common sites. Pyoderma may complicate scabies, onchocerciasis or other infestations, and contact or other forms of dermatitis.

Diagnosis is based on the clinical picture of mixed lesions, and isolation and culture of the organisms from the lesions.

Pyoderma should be treated with appropriate systemic antibiotics determined by antibiotic sensitivity tests.

Any underlying dermatosis or systemic disease should also be treated.

3.11 Gangrene

Necrosis or death of circumscribed parts of the skin may follow some severe infections, septicaemia or leukaemia.

In children, gangrene may follow severe infectious fevers such as varicella (chickenpox) and measles, or protein calorie malnutrition or

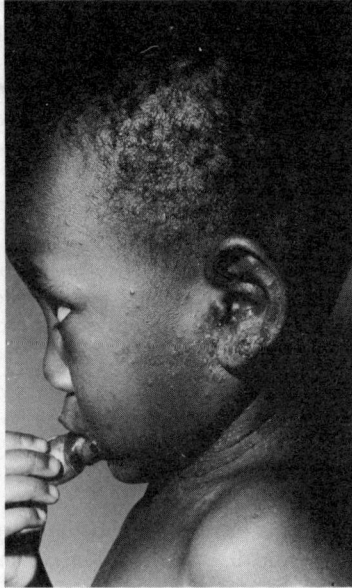

Figure 3.7 Pyoderma: impetigo, otitis externa and pustules on face and neck.

any debilitating illness. Cancrum oris is a most disfiguring form of gangrene.

In adults or children, gangrene may follow pyoderma, *Pseudomonas pyocyanea* infection, genital ulceration, or post-operative wound infections.

Diagnosis is based on the clinical nature and underlying disease, bacteriological examination of swabs and antibiotic sensitivity tests.

Treatment should be with antibiotics as determined by antibiotic sensitivity tests.

If gangrenous tissue is extensive, surgical excision may be necessary. Any underlying systemic disease should be treated.

3.12 Tropical ulcer

This develops from a small injury (cut, scratch, prick or insect bite) which becomes infected and necrotic, and grows rapidly into a foul-smelling crater with raised or undermined edges. The lower legs and feet are the commonest sites (plate 3). The affected part is usually painful.

The condition is commonest in children and young adults especially those exposed by their work to frequent trauma in the farms or fields. Poor hygiene, poverty and protein calorie malnutrition are among the predisposing factors. Hot humid climates also favour the development of tropical ulcer.

Treatment

Medical management The leg should be rested and may need to be elevated. The ulcer should be cleansed with hydrogen peroxide, potassium permanganate solution, eusol or Acriflavine.

Antibiotics should be given systematically and pain relieved with analgesics.

Surgical management After good granulation tissue has developed, skin grafting of the ulcer may be necessary.

3.13 Anthrax

This is a life-threatening acute infection caused by *Bacillus anthracis*. It is a disease of domestic animals such as cattle, horses, goats and sheep and human infection is usually seen in people handling live animals or their products.

Clinical features

Following infection with the bacillus, a dusky papule develops and ruptures within a few days. The underlying tissue is black and necrotic. Oedema of the surrounding area develops and lymphangitis, regional lymphadenitis and septicaemia follow rapidly. Constitutional symptoms include fever, toxaemia, prostration and collapse.

The mortality in untreated cases is high.

Diagnosis is based on the clinical picture, isolation of *Bacillus anthracis* in smears, cultures and blood culture, and by animal inoculation.

Treatment

Penicillin G 800,000 units–1.2 megaunits daily for 7–10 days should be given. Chlortetracycline 2 g daily in divided doses is also effective.

In advanced cases intravenous infusion should be set up and corticosteroids may be required.

4 Leprosy (Hansen's Disease)

Leprosy is a chronic infectious disease of man, and man has been aware of it for many centuries. A lot is known about leprosy, but ignorance also abounds concerning its nature, features, treatment, prognosis and control possibilities.

The disease was once global in distribution but is now confined largely to Asia, Africa and South America.

Leprosy bacilli attack mainly peripheral nerves, skin and mucosa of the upper respiratory tract. The clinical manifestations of the disease depend on the body's immune response to the presence of the bacilli. If the immune response is poor, the more severe or infectious type of disease (lepromatous leprosy) develops. If the immune response is good, the milder and much commoner 'non-infectious' type of disease (tuberculoid leprosy) develops.

Leprosy can be diagnosed fairly easily. It is amenable to treatment especially if the diagnosis is made early. With care and dedication in the application of the available diagnostic, therapeutic and control methods, the incidence can be drastically reduced in the developing world where the disease is now concentrated.

Leprosy is caused by the lepra bacillus (*Mycobacterium leprae*). It is usually characterised by a long incubation period, a prolonged clinical course, and predominant involvement of peripheral nerves, skin and mucous membrane of the upper respiratory tract.

In more severe infections, muscles, tendons, bones, the reticulo-endothelial system, testes and other viscera may be involved.

Partly because of facial and limb deformities which may follow untreated or badly treated cases, leprosy tends to invoke in man dread and horror to a degree that no other disease does. Such reactions are unfortunate and unjustified since the disease is amenable to treatment, and deformities are preventable, not inevitable.

Leprosy has been known to man for many centuries. References have been made to it in ancient Chinese, Indian and Hebrew literature. It remains a disease of under-development. The World Health Organization Expert Committee on Leprosy 1977 estimated that the total number of leprosy cases in the world would exceed twelve million (*WHO Technical Report Series* 607). About 95 per cent of these cases are to be found in Asia, Africa and South America. It is therefore, in these parts that the challenge to control the disease should be taken up with the fervour of a crusade.

4.1   'Types' of leprosy

Leprosy is a single disease, but there are two main clinical pictures of this disease: *tuberculoid leprosy* and *lepromatous leprosy*.

Tuberculoid leprosy is much commoner, less infectious and more readily amenable to treatment. The skin lesions are usually few in number, pale in colour, flat and insensitive to touch.

Lepromatous leprosy is less common, more infectious and more difficult to treat. The skin lesions are usually widespread, dusky, thickened and may or may not be insensitive to touch.

Leprosy is however properly classified into five 'types', based on clinical features, bacteriological examination, immunological reaction and histopathological picture. The clinical features reflect pathological changes which depend on the body's cell mediated immune response to the presence of lepra bacilli in the body.

  (1) Polar 'types':
      (a) Tuberculoid leprosy (TT) (figures 4.1 and 4.2 and plate 4)
      (b) Lepromatous leprosy (LL) (figure 4.3 and plates 5 and 6)
  (2) Intermediate 'types':
      (a) Borderline tuberculoid leprosy (BT)
      (b) Borderline leprosy (BB)
      (c) Borderline lepromatous leprosy (BL)

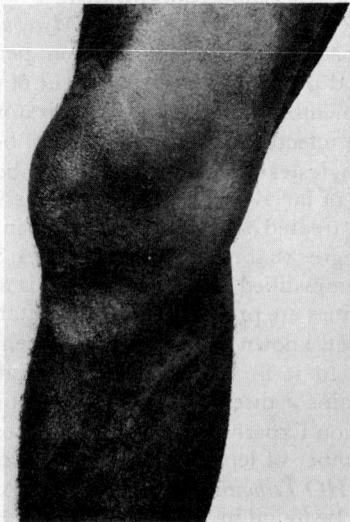

Figure 4.1   Tuberculoid leprosy: anaesthetic pale macule on medial aspect of knee and thigh.

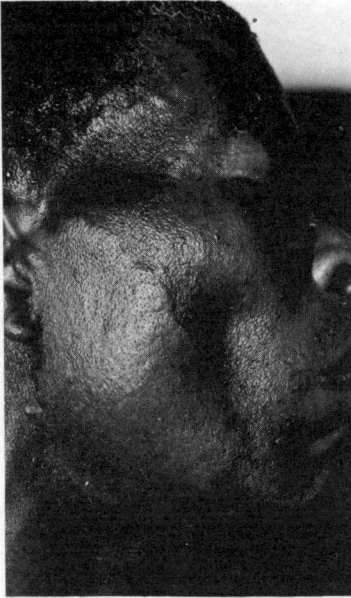

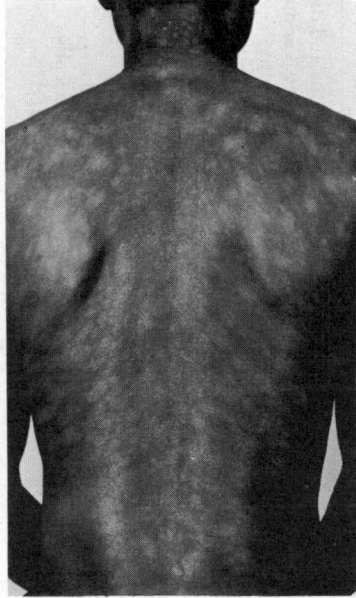

Figure 4.2   *(Left)* Tuberculoid leprosy: raised plaque on cheek.
Figure 4.3   *(Right)* Diffuse macular lepromatous leprosy.

Two polar 'types' (TT and LL) represent the ends of a wide spectrum of immunological response of the body to the presence of lepra bacilli in the body; while the intermediate 'types' BT, BB and BL represent various intermediate points on this spectrum between TT and LL. The main features of the different 'types' are summarised in table 4.1.

4.2 Pathology

The target organ of *M. leprae* is the peripheral nerve. On entering the body via the skin or mucosa, the bacilli reach the peripheral nerves and are soon found in the Schwann cells. Thereafter, their multiplication or destruction and the clinical picture of the disease produced depend on the cell-mediated immune response of the body (figure 4.4).

4.3 Epidemiology

Children and adolescents are more prone to the disease than adults.

Table 4.1 Main Features in Different Types of Leprosy

Features	TT	BT	BB	BL	LL
Number of skin lesions	One or few	Few	Many	Numerous	Numerous and diffuse
Size	2 cm–20 cm or more	Variable	Variable	Extensive	Widespread nodules
Colour	Pale	Pale	Dull or dusky	Dusky	Dusky, shiny
Symmetry	Not symmetrical	Not symmetrical	Tendency to symmetry	Tendency to symmetry	Symmetrical
Margin	Distinct	Distinct	Mixed, distinct and blurred	Tendency to be diffuse	Diffuse
Thickness	Flat early lesions. Raised older lesions	Raised and flat in parts	Flat or raised	Distinct papules	Thick nodules
Sensation to touch	Impaired	Impaired	Impaired	Impaired but not symmetrically	Impaired symmetrically
Sensation to temperature	Impaired	Variable	Impaired	Impaired	Impaired
Sweating	Impaired	Impaired	Impaired	Impaired	Impaired
Peripheral nerves	Thickened	Thickened	Thickened but asymmetrical	Thickened but asymmetrical	Thickened symmetrically
Nerve damage	Early	Early	Severe	Slow	Slow, diffuse
Lepra reaction	Possible	Common	Possible	Common	Common
Paresis	Early	Early	Severe	Slow	Slow, diffuse
Trophic ulcers	Common but avoidable	Uncommon	Possible	Possible	Common
Multiple organs	No	No	Rare	Mucosa	Nose, larynx, eyes, bones, testes
Facial deformity	No	No	No	Possible	Yes
Blindness	No	No	No	Possible	Yes
Bacilli in lesions	No	No	Scanty	Many	Numerous
Cell-mediated immunity	Very high	High	Average	Low	Nil
Lepromin test	Positive	Positive	Variable	Negative	Negative
Histology	Tuberculoid	Tuberculoid	Mixed picture	Tendency to lepromatous	Lepromatous

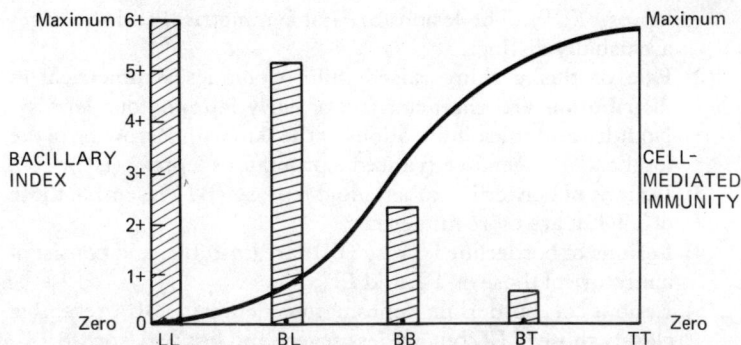

Figure 4.4   Inverse relationship between cell-mediated immunity and bacillary index.

Most infections are established in childhood even though the diagnosis may be made in adult life. The rate of spread of the disease in a community depends on the proportion of susceptible individuals and the chances of contact with infectious cases, usually the lepromatous LL and borderline lepromatous BL cases.

4.4 **Diagnosis**

A careful clinical examination for skin lesions, anaesthesia, and thickened nerves followed by examination of slit skin and nasal mucosal smears for lepra bacilli will usually be sufficient to make a diagnosis.

Important points to ask about in the history before or while conducting the clinical examination include: numbness, pale flat or raised skin lesions, difficulty in holding objects, difficulty in walking, painlessness of recent burns or injuries, and eye trouble. It is also necessary to ask for previous treatment with dapsone and, more tactfully, for family contact with leprosy. Family contact is not very readily admitted for the obvious reason of fear of the stigma.

Clinical examination

The cardinal signs are skin lesions, anaesthesia and thickened nerves. Lepra bacilli should then be looked for.

Skin lesions

   (1) Pale macules or raised plaques are characteristic of tuberculoid

leprosy (TT). The lesions are not symmetrical and the edges are usually distinct.

(2) Pale or dusky shiny raised diffuse plaques symmetrical in distribution are characteristic of early lepromatous leprosy. Nodules and thick infiltrations of the skin with furrowing of the forehead are seen in advanced lepromatous leprosy (LL).

(3) Lesions of borderline tuberculoid leprosy (BT) resemble those of TT but are more numerous.

(4) Lesions of borderline leprosy (BB) are unstable, and consist of a mixture of those or TT and LL.

(5) Lesions of borderline lepromatous leprosy (BL) resemble closely those of LL but are less severe and less widespread.

(6) Indeterminate leprosy: symptomless ill-defined pale macules which have not developed features determinate of their position on some point of the TT–LL spectrum may be seen on the face or trunk or limbs. They are classified as indeterminate and should be watched carefully for a change to any of the other types.

Anaesthesia A wisp of cotton wool or a piece of paper may be used to touch various points on the pale patch or raised plaque or surrounding area. Demonstrate the test to the patient looking before asking him to close his eyes and then touch with his index finger any points on his body which you may touch subsequently.

In TT and BT the sensation of touch is impaired or lost over the pale macules or raised plaques and over the distribution of the thickened peripheral nerves.

In LL and BL the sensation is impaired more extensively especially on the extensor surfaces of the hands, forearms, feet and legs.

In BB, the sensation is also impaired early but more in relation to the lesions.

In indeterminate leprosy, the sensation may be normal or only slightly impaired over the pale macules.

Two test tubes filled with hot water and cold water may also be used to test for impairment of temperature sensation over the affected areas.

Thickened nerves Peripheral nerves which are commonly thickened in leprosy especially in tuberculoid leprosy (TT) are the ulnar, posterior tibial, lateral popliteal or peroneal, great auricular, supra-orbital and radial nerve at the wrist. These nerves should be palpated while examining a patient.

Thickening of nerves usually precedes signs of nerve damage. In lepra reactions, however, thickening, tenderness and paresis appear together with other signs of the reaction, for example, nodules, fever, and joint pains.

Examination for lepra bacilli (acid fast bacilli) Slit skin smears from macules, plaques, nodules or diffuse skin thickening and nasal muco-sal smears or nose blow smears should be made on microscope slides and examined by the Ziehl-Neelsen method. Bacilli are seen in greatest concentrations in lepromatous leprosy (LL). The concentration falls gradually in BL, BB and BT. Usually no bacilli are seen in tuberculoid leprosy TT or in indeterminate leprosy.

Bacillary index and morphological index The concentration or density of bacilli in an average field in the microscope slide is graded from 6+ to 0. This is the bacillary index.

Some bacilli are solid staining (*living*) while others stain irregularly or are fragmented (*dead*).

The percentage of solid staining bacilli is the morphological index. It is about 50 in lepromatous leprosy at the beginning of treatment.

The rate of fall of the morphological index during treatment is an indication of the effectiveness of the drug in use.

Lepromin test Lepromin is a crude extract of bacilli from a lepromatous nodule. Lepromin (0.1 ml) is injected into the skin (forearm or upper arm) and the site is examined at 72 hours and 3–4 weeks for a palpable nodule. The test is not used for diagnosis but is an indication of delayed hypersensitivity to lepra bacilli antigens. The test is strongly positive in TT and positive in BT. It is negative in LL and BL and is doubtful in BB.

The early positive reaction is the Fernandez reaction showing erythema and induration after about 72 hours.

The late positive reaction is the Mitsuda reaction showing a palpable nodule after 3–4 weeks.

Blood tests In lepromatous LL and borderline lepromatous BL cases, anaemia may be found. False positive tests for lupus erythematosus cells and syphilis may also be found.

Systemic complications In the absence of cell mediated immune re-sponse, severe infection may involve the reticulo-endothelial system, haemopoietic system, bones, testes, muscles. Death may occur from intercurrent infection such as tuberculosis, or from amyloidosis or anaemia.

4.5   **Treatment of leprosy**

The first thing to know about leprosy is that it is treatable. This fact should be conveyed to the patient and to his relatives at the very beginning.

Sulphones

Diaminodiphenyl sulphone (dapsone, DDS, Avlosulphone) remains the front line drug for routine treatment. It is usually given by mouth.

Action Dapsone is bacteriostatic, interfering with the metabolism of lepra bacilli. It can bring the morphological index in lepromatous leprosy down to zero in 6–12 months.

Dosage 50–100 mg (tablets) daily in adults.
     25–50 mg daily in children.
   Dapsone injections can be given in doses of 600 mg i.m. weekly or 300–400 mg twice weekly.

Duration of treatment This should be until no signs of disease activity are detectable. In TT, this should be achieved in about 3 years; in BT and BB in about 5–8 years; and in BL and LL in 10 years or more.

Drawbacks Side effects include haemolytic anaemia, agranulocytosis, fixed drug eruption, other allergic eruptions, lepra reactions, and psychotic reactions.
   The emergence of dapsone-resistant lepra bacilli has been reported. This leads to relapses during treatment and reappearance of solid staining bacilli.

Combined treatment

Dapsone is very cheap. Other effective drugs are very expensive. Severity of the disease, the appearance of dapsone resistance, or erythema nodosum leprosum or reversal reaction may call for combined treatment.

Dapsone plus clofazimine
   Dapsone 50–100 mg daily   }
   Clofazimine 100 mg daily   } for 4–6 months
   Followed by dapsone 50–100 mg daily.

Dapsone plus rifampicin
 Dapsone 50–100mg daily ⎱ for 4 weeks
 Rifampicin 600mg daily ⎰
 Followed by dapsone 50–100 mg daily.

Clofazimine plus rifampicin
 In proven dapsone-resistant cases,
 Clofazimine 100 mg daily ⎱ for 3 months
 Rifampicin 600 mg daily ⎰
 Followed by clofazimine 100 mg daily.

Treatment of severe lepra reactions

Reversal reactions with severe nerve damage, or erythema nodosum leprosum with tender nodules, thickened nerves, fever and general malaise, joint pains, eye involvement, proteinuria and orchitis call for clofazimine, analgesics and prednisolone. Clofazimine can be given in increased doses of 200–300 mg daily and prednisolone at 20 mg t.i.d. gradually tailed off.

Drawbacks of clofazimine and rifampicin

Clofazimine has the drawback of excessive darkening of the skin and can scarcely be accepted by the patient for more than three months. It may also cause diarrhoea in some patients.
 Rifampicin is bacteriocidal and can bring the morphological index down to zero in 4–6 weeks but is very expensive and has the side effects of haemolytic anaemia, thrombocytopenia and fever.

Thiambutosine (*Diphenyl thiourea*: CIBA 1906)

This drug is bacteriostatic, as effective as dapsone and free of toxic effects, but lepra bacilli develop resistance to it readily. It is useful in initiating treatment in patients with borderline leprosy and a tendency to lepra reactions.

4.6 Leprosy control

'If existing knowledge about leprosy were conscientiously and persistently applied, the disease could be CONTROLLED IN THIS GENERATION, and eradicated in the next' – Dr Stanley G. Browne, 1971.
 Unfortunately those parts of the world which need to adopt a

crusading spirit against leprosy in their midst so that the above prophecy can come true are definitely not yet doing the best they can.

The objectives of leprosy control

These include:
  (1) To reduce the infection in the human reservoir by effective chemotherapy.
  (2) To provide prompt and adequate early treatment for all diagnosed cases, thereby avoiding the disabling and disheartening complications and deformities.
  (3) To protect the healthy population.

The main elements of a leprosy control programme

These are:
  (1) Prompt and adequate drug treatment of individual patients.
  (2) Re-education of doctors, nurses and other health workers to rid them of their fears of an ordinary disease which many of them still erroneously consider extraordinary.
  (3) Mobilisation of the community for a community effort in leprosy control and control of other prevalent diseases.
  (4) Estimation of prevalence of leprosy by means of epidemiological surveys of high risk groups, institutions and whole populations.
  (5) Case detection in rural areas and in urban areas.
  (6) Contact surveillance of households with lepromatous cases.
  (7) Raising the general standard of living and hygiene.
  (8) Control methods which are complementary to drug treatment
    (a) Hospitalisation of patients who require intensive surgical, ophthalmic or special care.
    (b) Occupational and social rehabilitation.
  (9) Control measures which are still at the experimental stage
    (a) BCG vaccination of household contacts, children and other high risk groups.
    (b) Dapsone prophylaxis for special high risk groups.
    (c) Specific vaccination with vaccines produced from lepra bacilli inoculated into armadillos.

5 Infestations by Animal Parasites

The environment and the quality of life determine the incidence of infestations by animal parasites. These infestations are most prevalent in unhygienic home environments and rural work environments such as farms, forests and markets.

Scabies, lice, bedbugs, jiggers and fleas share the homes while various larvae infest the surrounding compounds or gardens, the insect vectors of filarial worms inhabit farms, bushes and forests, and the carriers of guinea worm make well and pond water unsafe. The skin diseases caused by these animal parasites can all be treated, but it is far better and cheaper in the long run to improve the standard of personal and home hygiene, to attempt to control the habitats of the known carriers of the other diseases, and to provide safe drinking water free of the carriers of guinea worm and other diseases.

The skin can be attacked by many types of insects, bugs, larvae and worms. Bites or stings by these animal parasites or their presence in the skin may produce various distinct clinical patterns or may even cause systemic illness.

The common infestations include scabies, various forms of filariasis, pediculosis (lice), dracontiasis (guinea worm), larva migrans (creeping eruption), cutaneous myiasis (tumbu fly), jiggers, bedbug bites and flea bites.

5.1 Scabies

This is a contagious disease caused by the itch mite, *Sarcoptes scabiei*. It is accompanied by marked itching especially at night.

Scabies is usually transmitted by close personal contact. The warm closeness and low standard of hygiene in large families, schools, barracks, camps, prisons etc. favour the spread of the disease. The overcrowding imposed by war conditions and natural disasters also causes an increase in incidence of the disease. Many members of a family or close-living group may suffer from the disease at the same time. Scabies may also be sexually transmitted.

Natural history of scabies

Following the infestation of a new host by fertilised females or nymphs, the mites burrow into the horny layer of the epidermis. The pregnant females lay eggs in the burrows while the nymphs moult about three times to develop into adult mites within two weeks. The new eggs hatch in 3–4 days, nymphs emerging to start their moulting.

Adult male mites usually die soon after fertilising the females while the adult females die after they have laid about 20 eggs over a period of 10–14 days. But the disease continues since relays of eggs, nymphs and adults are around to maintain the infestation.

Itching usually starts in an infested host after about two weeks as an allergic reaction to the mites and their products. In subsequent infestations, itching may start only a few days after, indicating that the individual had been sensitised by an earlier infestation.

In a rare form of scabies described as 'crusted scabies' or 'Norwegian scabies', the normal reaction of itching is absent in the patient either because of mental illness or neurological disorder. The infestation by scabies therefore becomes extensive or generalised with thickening, scaling and crusting of the skin which teems with mites.

Common sites and characterictic lesions (figures 5.1–5.3)

The mites prefer the hidden and furrowed sites from where they cannot easily be scratched off. These sites include the webs and sides of the fingers, wrists and ulnar border of the hands, elbows, axillary folds, areola of the breasts, umbilicus, waist, external genitalia and perineum, natal cleft, thighs, knees and ankles. In children, the palms and soles may also be affected.

The characteristic primary lesions found in these sites are papules and runs or burrows. Runs or burrows are short wavy papular eruptions overlying the burrows harbouring the mites, eggs, nymphs, excreta and debris.

Vesicles, bullae, pustules, nodules, impetiginised lesions, eczematised lesions, crusts, scabs, erosions and excoriations may complicate the papules and burrows.

Complications of scabies

Secondary bacterial infection. Staphylococcal or streptococcal infection may complicate scabies and lead to pyoderma, cellulitis, lymphangitis, lymphadenitis or even septicaemia and glomerulonephritis.

Eczema or dermatitis. Wrong diagnosis and treatment with irritant applications may provoke a dermatitis.

Acarophobia. Long after the infestation has been cleared, a few patients may develop this psychiatric complication, a delusion that the skin is infested with scabies.

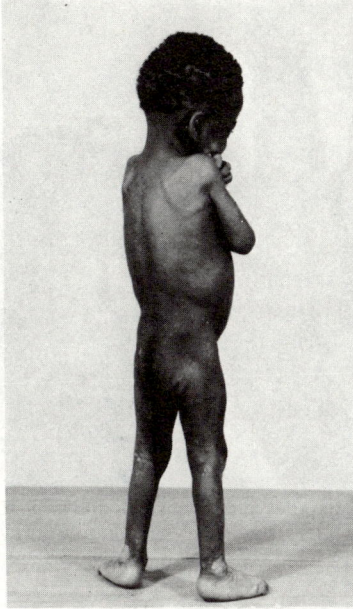

Figure 5.1   Scabies: child with widespread scabies in skin folds, scratching away in misery.

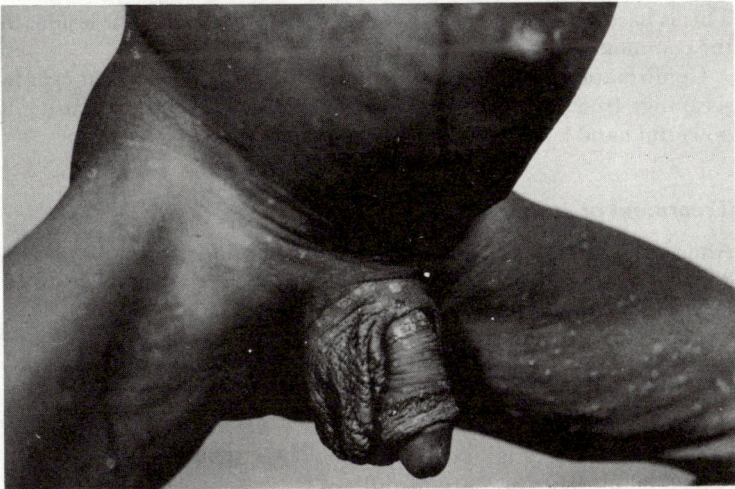

Figure 5.2   Scabies: same child with papules and scratch marks around the waist, inner thighs and external genitalia.

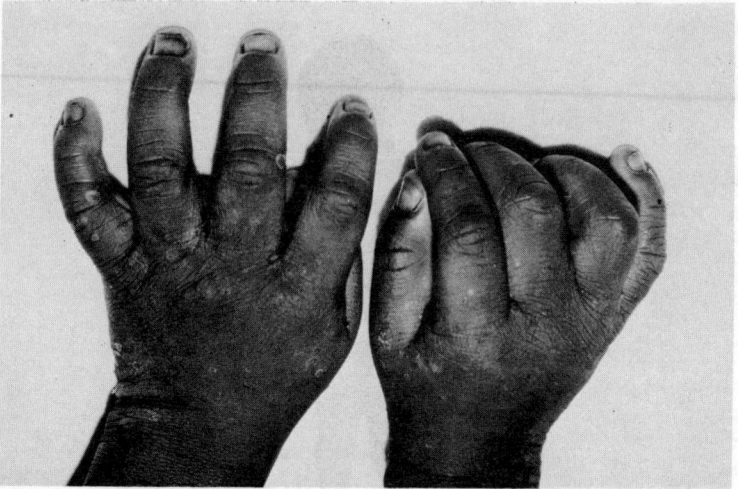

Figure 5.3   Scabies: papules, burrows, scabs and crusts in the webs of the
fingers and on the wrists.

Diagnosis of scabies

This is based on the history and the finding of characteristic lesions in
the common sites.

Confirmation rests with the demonstration of the acarus or eggs in
scrapings from the burrows or crusts examined on a slide using a
powerful hand lens or the low power of a microscope.

Treatment of scabies

After a thorough bath, scrubbing with soap and sponge followed by
drying of the skin, 25 per cent benzyl benzoate emulsion is rubbed
well into the skin from the neck down to the toes.

All affected members of the family should be treated at the same
time and the procedure should be repeated on two or three successive
nights.

Antihistamines should be given for the relief of itching.

Secondary bacterial infection should be treated with systemic
penicillin or other appropriate antibiotic.

Other useful scabicides include Ascabiol (benzyl benzoate), Eurax
(crotamiton) and monosulphiram (Tetmosol).

5.2   **Filarial infestations**

There are three main filarial worms (nematodes) which cause filarial infestations. They are transmitted by insect vectors.

Nematode	Insect vector	Disease	Principal organs/system
Onchocerca volvulus	*Simulium* (black flies)	Onchocerciasis	Skin, eyes
Filaria loa	*Chrysops* (mangrove flies)	Loaiasis (Calabar swellings)	Skin, eyes
Wuchereria bancrofti *Brugia malayi*	Mosquitoes (various species)	Filariasis (elephantiasis)	Lymphatics

5.3   **Onchocerciasis** *(river blindness)*

This is a filarial disease caused by *Onchocerca volvulus*, a nematode transmitted by black flies of the genus Simulidae. In Africa, *Simulium damnosum* is the common vector.

The disease is found in a wide belt stretching from West Africa across Central and East Africa to the Middle East. It is also found in Central and South America.

Natural history of onchocerciasis

Nodular stage Following bites by infected black flies, microfilariae injected into the dermis become walled off by fibrous tissue reactions. Over a period of 6–9 months, these microfilariae develop into adult worms within fibrous capsules which are visible and palpable near bony prominences around the waist, ribs or shoulders or on the scalp. These are onchocerca nodules or onchocercomata.

Eruptive stage (figures 5.4–5.6) Within the nodules, adult male and female worms copulate, the males die off and the gravid females lay eggs which hatch into a new crop of microfilariae.

These microfilariae migrate from the nodules into surrounding tissues producing a train of pruritic eruptions: urticaria, papules,

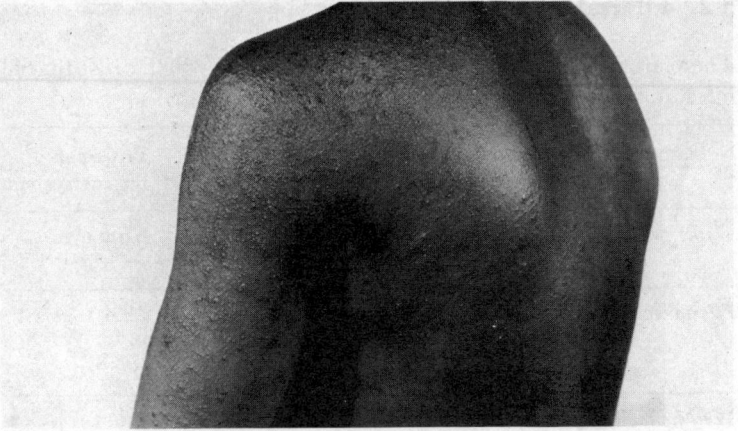

Figure 5.4   Onchodermatitis: eruptive stage. Widespread distribution of papules, wheals, scratch marks, thickened and hyperpigmented skin on affected side of the body.

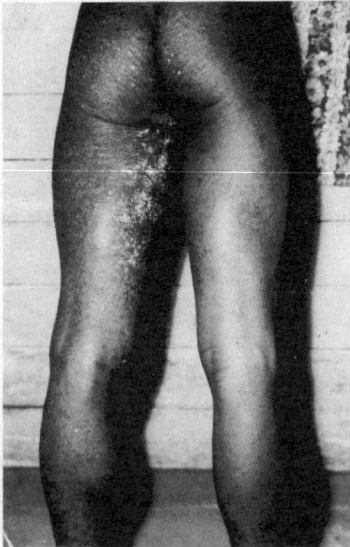

Figure 5.5   *(Left)* Onchodermatitis: lesions still more profuse on one side in advanced stage.

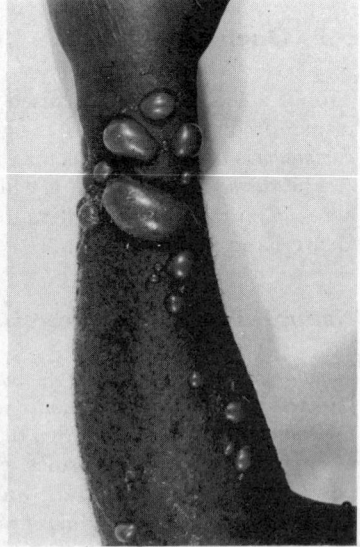

Figure 5.6   *(Right)* Onchodermatitis: swelling of the arm with vesicles and bullae. Mazzotti reaction to treatment with diethylcarbamazine (Banocide).

nodules and vesicles. Cellulitis, lymphangitis, lymphadenitis and lymphoedema may also develop. Scratching will also lead to the development of excoriations, pustules, induration, lichenification and hyperpigmentation.

There is a tendency for the lesions of onchocerciasis to be related to the site of the nodules. The eruptions are therefore usually unilateral in the early stages and even when they are widespread, one side of the body tends to be more severely involved than the opposite side.

Ocular lesions In regions where the vectors tend to bite on the head, neck or upper trunk, microfilariae in the eruptive stage invade the eye and cause keratitis, choroiditis and uveitis which can lead to impaired vision or even blindness (river blindness).

Chronic stage (figures 5.7–5.9) After many years without treatment, atrophic and fibrotic changes in the skin and subcutaneous tissues may lead to depigmentary changes on the shins, thighs and over bony prominences, hanging groins, verrucosity, elephantiasis, and calcification of onchocerca nodules.

Diagnosis of onchocerciasis

   (1) Demonstration of adult worms in excised onchocerca nodules.
   (2) Demonstration of microfilariae in teased out skin snips.

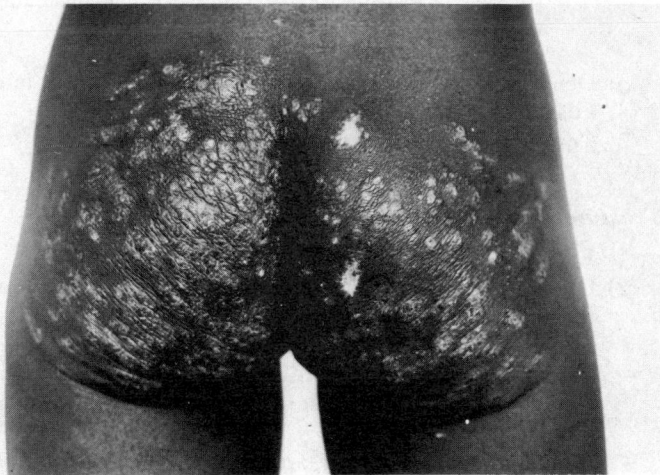

Figure 5.7   Onchodermatitis: skin induration, lichenified plaques and mottled hypopigmentation.

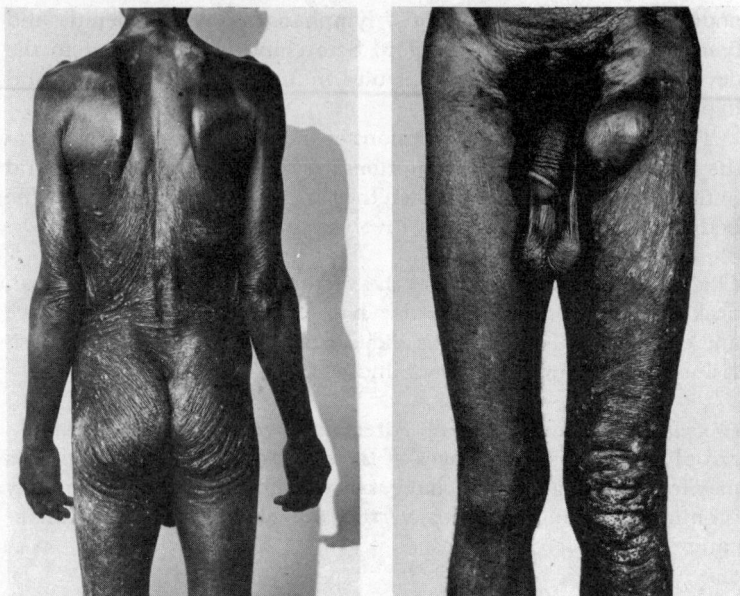

Figure 5.8   *(Left)* Onchodermatitis: very advanced stage with skin atrophy and mottled hypopigmentation.

Figure 5.9   *(Right)* Onchodermatitis: very advanced stage with skin atrophy (in parts), thickening (in parts) mottled hypopigmentation and regional lymphadenopathy.

(3) Demonstration of microfilariae in the eyes, using slit lamp.
(4) Filarial skin test.
(5) Complement fixation test.

Treatment of onchocerciasis

(1) Excision of onchocerca nodules.
(2) Diethylcarbamazine citrate (Banocide) is very effective against the microfilariae. Dosage should be low initially 25–50 mg t.i.d. to avoid severe reactions (Mazzotti reaction). The dosage should be increased at monthly intervals up to a maximum of 75–150 mg t.i.d. The course of treatment is usually 6 months or more for effective cure.

   For the relief of itching, antihistamines by mouth and antihistamine lotion or cream or calamine lotion or cream topically are useful.

(3) Suramin (Antrypol) is effective against the adult worms, but it is nephrotoxic, and the urine should be examined weekly for protein, red cells and casts before the drug is given.

The course of treatment is 0.5 g intravenously weekly for 4–6 weeks.

Control of onchocerciasis

Control of the vectors is effected by clearing bushes or spraying their breeding sites with insecticides.

5.4 Loaiasis *(loa loa, Calabar swellings)*

This is filarial infestation caused by another nematode, *Filaria loa* transmitted by the insect vector *Chrysops* spp. (red mangrove flies) which bite by day and pick up from or inject into man the microfilariae of *Filaria loa*. Loaiasis is common in the rain forest belt of West Africa.

Natural history of loaiasis

Maturation Following the bite by an infected *Chrysops*, the microfilariae develop in the dermis or subcutaneous tissues into adult worms over a period of 6–12 months.

Migratory stage Adult worms wander about through the subcutaneous tissues, provoking transient large urticarial swellings on various parts of the body. If the eye is involved, oedema of the eyelids develops, and the worm may be seen under the conjunctiva. Filarial worms may also cause joint swellings.

Burnt-out stage After some years, the adult worms may die and calcify in the subcutaneous tissue.

Diagnosis

(1) Migratory urticarial or oedematous swellings, itchy or painful in a patient from an endemic area.
(2) Demonstration of microfilariae in blood taken by day.
(3) Filarial skin test.
(4) Complement fixation test.

Treatment

Diethylcarbamazine is effective and should be given in the same graded dose for about one month.

5.5 **Elephantiasis** *(Bancroftian filariasis)*

This is another filarial infestation, caused by *Wuchereria bancrofti* or *Brugia malayi* whose vectors are night-biting *Culex, Anopheles* or *Aedes* mosquitoes.

It is a disease of the tropical and subtropical regions stretching from Central and South America, tropical Africa, the Mediterranean region, Middle East, India and the Far East and Northern Australia.

Natural history of elephantiasis

Early lymphatic phase Following the bite by infected mosquitoes, microfilariae invade the lymphatics and lymph nodes. Adult worms develop in lymphatic vessels over a period of about one year. There may or may not be bouts of fever, lymphangitis and lymphadenitis.

Stage of filarial fevers Adult female worms produce microfilariae which invade the lymphatics and blood and produce frequent bouts of fever, cellulitis, lymphangitis, and lymphadenitis. Microfilariae can be demonstrated in peripheral blood taken at night.

Stage of elephantiasis This may develop slowly over a period of years or may be precipitated by severe constitutional upset characterised by erythema, urticaria, lymphangitis, lymphadenitis, epididymo-orchitis and scrotal swelling. Elephantiasis usually involves the scrotum or labia and the lower legs. Occasionally the arms or breasts may become affected. The overlying skin is indurated and verrucose.

Diagnosis

Usually obvious clinically. Microfilariae may be demonstrated in the blood at night and adult worms in the tissues.

Treatment

Medical: diethylcarbamazine as in onchocerccasis.
Surgical: plastic repair of redundant tissues.

5.6 **Dracontiasis** *(Guinea worm)*

This is an infestation by a nematode *Dracunculus medinensis* transmitted through the ingestion of water fleas of the genus *Cyclops* found in wells or stagnant water.

It is a disease of underdevelopment, found in Africa, the Middle East, Asia and the Far East.

Natural history of dracontiasis

Gastrointestinal stage Following the ingestion of the *Cyclops* in water, gastric juice digests the *Cyclops* and the nematode larvae are released.

Retroperitoneal stage The larvae penetrate the intestinal wall into the retroperitoneal space where they develop into adult worms in 6–12 months. They copulate, the males die off and the gravid females continue their migration to dependent parts of the body usually the lower legs.

Subcutaneous stage In the subcutaneous tissue of the legs, feet or other parts, the gravid female bulging with larvae penetrates the skin and protrudes through an indurated area or blister which soon ulcerates. It pours out thousands of motile larvae into the opening which usually comes into contact with water (plate 7).

Cyclops stage Motile larvae can survive for a few days in the water until they are ingested by *Cyclops* in which they complete their development into a stage infective to man.

Clinical features

Only during the migration of the gravid female worm in the subcutaneous tissue is the infestation evident. There may be urticaria, cellulitis, lymphangitis, lymphadenitis and fever.

The blister and ulcer are accompanied by induration and painful swelling of the affected limb. Chronic ulcers may develop.

Complications associated with lesions around joints may include arthritis and ankylosis.

Tetanus is a possible danger should the ulcer become contaminated with soil.

Treatment of dracontiasis

Diethylcarbamazine is effective against the worm before it has penetrated to the subcutaneous tissue but not after that. When the adult worm has emerged from a broken vesicle or bulla, mechanical extraction of the worm by slowly winding it on a match-stick may help to extract it completely. It may however break, and cellulitis and induration of the surrounding skin may develop.

Antibiotics and antihistamines are helpful in combating cellulitis and allergic reactions.

Prophylaxis Improvement in supply of drinking water and the boiling and filtering of drinking water will prevent the disease.

5.7   **Pediculosis** *(lice infestation)*

Lice infestation may affect the scalp (pediculosis capitis), the body (pediculosis corporis) or the pubic region (pediculosis pubis). Lice infestation is much more prevalent than hospital figures may suggest since self medication is usually undertaken by most patients who are conscious of the stigma of uncleanliness associated with pediculosis.

Two species of lice (*Pediculus humanus* and *Phthirus pubis*) infest man. *Pediculus humanus capitis* causes pediculosis capitis, *Pediculus humanus corporis* causes pediculosis corporis while *Phthirus pubis* causes pediculosis pubis.

Itching and secondary bacterial infection are the main features of all lice infestations.

Pediculosis capitis

Head lice are usually confined to the scalp, and feed on blood. They may also invade the eyebrows, eye lashes and beard. They are transmitted by body contact and the sharing of head gear and fomites. Pruritus is the main symptom of pediculosis.

The adult females lay their eggs (nits) which are attached to the hair shafts. Secondary bacterial infection follows scratching and pyoderma, folliculitis, furunculosis, lymphangitis and occipital and cervical lymphadenitis may complicate the infestation.

Diagnosis This is based on the history of pruritus and the finding of greyish black adults or ovoid greyish nits, scalp infection and occipital or cervical lymphadenitis.

Effective scalp applications include

(1) Dichlorodiphenyltrichloroethane (DDT) emulsion 5 per cent;
(2) Gamma benzene hexachloride (BHC) shampoo and
(3) Malathion lotion 0.5 per cent.

Treatment Prior cutting of the hair is often necessary. Washing and combing of the hair to examine for lice and their nits. Treatment may be repeated if infestation persists. Pruritus should be treated with antihistamines and secondary bacterial infection with appropriate antibiotics.

Pediculosis corporis

Body lice usually live in the seams of clothing and crawl on to the body to suck blood. They are transmitted by clothing, bedding and other fomites. They provoke itching and the scratching is followed by secondary bacterial infection.

Diagnosis This is based on the history of pruritus, the finding of lice and nits on the seams of clothing and itchy eczematous eruptions or secondary bacterial infection on the trunk or limbs.

Treatment The clothing and bedding should be treated with DDT powder or benzene hexachloride (BHC) in talcum powder and washed thoroughly. The skin eruptions should be treated with calamine lotion and pruritus controlled with antihistamines.

Pediculosis pubis

Pubic lice usually invade the pubic region but may also be found on the lower abdomen, thighs, and even the axillae. They may be transmitted sexually, by close body contact or through clothes or fomites. Pediculosis pubis is often considered a sexually transmitted disease (see 18.9, p. 181).

Like head lice, pubic lice lay their eggs on hair shafts. They also suck blood, provoke itching and the resultant scratching leads to secondary bacterial infection and regional lymphadenitis.

Diagnosis This is based on the history of pubic or genital pruritus, the finding of lice and nits and eczematous eruptions or secondary bacterial infection.

Treatment Cutting of the hair and application of DDT emulsion, gamma benzene hexachloride (BHC), benzyl benzoate emulsion or malathion lotion as in pediculosis capitis.

5.8 Larva migrans *(creeping eruption)* (figure 5.10)

This is a tortuous thread-like inflammatory reaction on the skin produced by the larvae of various worms which get into the skin accidentally from contaminated soil or clothing. The larvae wander about in a 'blind alley' in the skin and never get out alive since skin infestation is not part of their natural cycle of development. Cat and dog hookworm larvae are among the common causes.

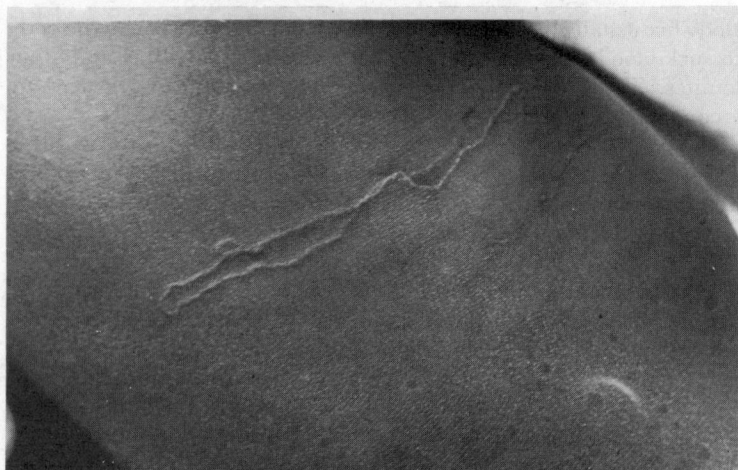

Figure 5.10   Cutaneous larva migrans (creeping eruption). Thread-like inflammatory reaction marking tortuous path of larva in the skin.

The inflammatory reaction may be accompanied by papules or vesicles and the tortuous course may be many centimetres long. Itching is severe and scratching may lead to secondary bacterial infection. The larvae may survive for some weeks before dying.

Treatment

Local treatment Freezing with ethyl chloride spray, carbon dioxide snow or liquid nitrogen is usually effective. Secondarily infected lesions may be treated with topical antibiotics.

Systemic treatment Thiabendazole 3–5 g orally weekly until larval activity ceases. Side effects of gastrointestinal upset and dizziness limit its routine use. In visceral larva migrans with lung involvement and hepatosplenomegaly and eosinophilia, the use of thiabendazole is appropriate.

5.9 **Tumbu fly** (figures 5.11 and 5.12)

In this form of cutaneous myiasis, the larvae of tumbu fly (*Cordylobia anthropophaga*) are picked up accidentally from contaminated soil or clothing.

The larvae attach themselves to the human skin, penetrate the skin, develop rapidly and produce painful boil-like swellings and surrounding cellulitis. They mature in one to two weeks, push their way out of the skin and drop to the ground to pupate.

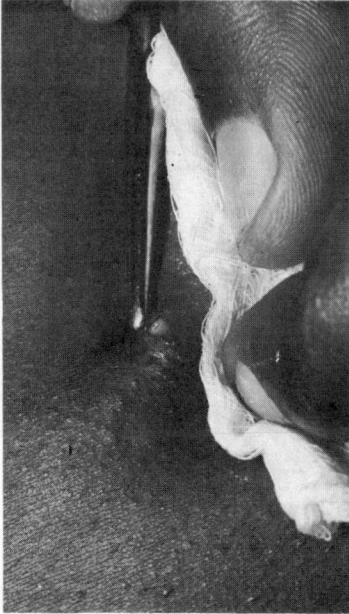

Figure 5.11   *(Left)* Tumbu fly: pustule with larva (maggot) in the skin.

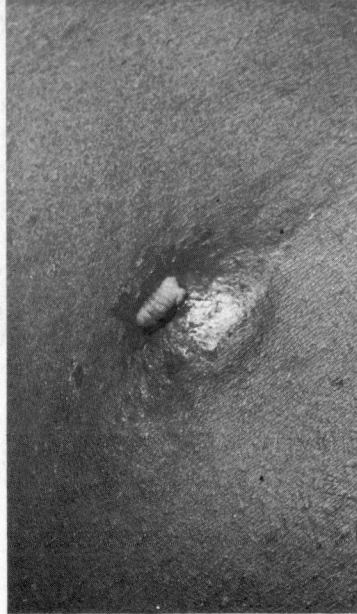

Figure 5.12   *(Right)* Tumbu fly: larva (maggot) expressed from pustule.

Diagnosis This is based on the history of painful 'boils' which fail to suppurate and on the horrifying discovery of maggots emerging from the 'boils'.

Treatment The maggots should be expressed and destroyed and the cellulitis treated with antibiotics.

5.9   Jiggers

The pregnant female of the sand flea (*Tunga penetrans*) attaches itself to the human toe or foot or other part of the body, burrows into the dermis and grows rapidly into a whitish maize seed-sized swelling which is largely uterus. It discharges eggs from its rear end near the skin surface until it dies.

The affected part of the toe or foot is swollen, painful and tender. Secondary bacterial infection, lymphangitis and lymphadenitis usually develop. The two dreaded complications of jigger infestation are septicaemia and tetanus.

Treatment

The jigger should be prised out as carefully as possible and destroyed. The cavity should be treated with antiseptics and secondary bacterial infection with antibiotics. A course of tetanus toxoid may be given.

5.10   Bedbug bites

These produce non-specific eczematous eruptions and secondary bacterial infections. The skin eruptions should be treated topically and measures to eradicate bedbugs adopted.

6 Fungal Infections

Spores of various fungi (simple plants) abound in the external environment. These get on to the skin or mucous membranes readily and, under favourable conditions, some germinate, grow and become pathogenic. Fungal infections may be superficial, affecting the skin, mucous membrane, hair and nails; or deep, affecting deeper structures and viscera.

Because fungal infections of the skin, hair, nails and mucosa are common and produce clinical pictures which resemble other diseases, there is a tendency to overdiagnose or misdiagnose fungal infections. Diagnosis of fungal infection should therefore be confirmed by demonstration and culture of the fungi from the lesions.

Tinea versicolor, common, classical in its scaliness and distribution in the upper trunk and cosmetically embarrassing, yields to confirmatory diagnosis by microscopic examination of scales from the lesion, and responds to prolonged application of appropriate keratolytic preparations.

The dermatophytes (fungi causing superficial skin infections) cause various infections ranging from tinea capitis to tinea pedis. They invade the horny layer of the skin, the hair or the nail. Their various species can be demonstrated microscopically and on culture. Dermatophytes respond to griseofulvin, an antifungal antibiotic.

Candida albicans, a yeast-like fungus can invade the mucosa, skin folds and nail folds, yields easily to demonstration and culture, and responds to nystatin (Mycostatin), clotrimazole (Canesten) and other fungicides.

Deep and visceral fungus infections mimic other diseases even more than superficial fungal infections do. They call for more ingenuity in diagnosis and expertise in management.

6.1 Superficial fungal infections

Fungi which cause superficial skin infections are called dermatophytes. They penetrate the top 1–2 mm of the epidermis where they digest and live on keratin. Superficial fungal infections are passed from person to person either directly or by indirect contact (clothing, footwear, household instruments, furniture). They can also be caught from infected domestic animals.

Common clinical types

Superficial fungal infections (tinea versicolor, ringworm, moniliasis) constitute 10–20% of skin diseases treated in hospitals.

6.2 **Pityriasis versicolor** (*tinea versicolor*) (plate 8)

This is a very common superficial fungal infection which presents as irregular macules or large confluent sheets of dry fine scales of various colours – brown, yellowish-brown, or dark brown – seen most commonly over the upper trunk, face, neck, shoulders and upper arms in teenagers and in young adults of both sexes. Masses of fungal hyphae and spores in the horny layer in the affected areas filter out actinic rays. These areas are therefore usually less tanned than the surrounding areas.

Tinea versicolor is cosmetically undesirable, but causes little or no itching. It tends to run a chronic course, and to recur after inadequate treatment.

It is caused by a fungus, *Malassezia furfur* which can be demonstrated microscopically in skin scrapings taken from the affected areas. *Malassezia furfur* appears as short hyphal elements (strands) and clusters of spores. It cannot be cultured yet. Wood's filtered ultraviolet light demonstrates the fluorescence of affected areas.

Treatment

Local applications which cause shedding of the horny layer of the epidermis along with the fungal spores and hyphae are effective, and should be used for 6–8 weeks. These include compound ointment of benzoic acid (Whitfield's ointment), salicylic acid ointment, sodium hyposulphite solution, and selenium sulphide suspension 2.5 per cent (Selsun)

Useful proprietary preparations are: tolnaftate solution; Canesten (clotrimazole) solution; Jadit solution (buclosamide + salicylic acid + hydrocortisone); H115 solution (chlormidazole hydrochloride + salicylic acid). Since tinea versicolor is resistant to treatment and reinfection is common, treatment should be persisted with for 6–8 weeks or more.

6.3 **Ringworm infections** (*tinea*)

These are caused by a variety of fungi (*Microsporum, Trichophyton* and *Epidermophyton*) and affect the skin, hair and nails.

Their spread is favoured by conditions of poor personal hygiene, heat and high humidity.

Immunological factors also play a part in determining the establishment and extent of fungal infections. Some individuals are more susceptible than others. Patients suffering from leukaemia or lymphoma and those on prolonged corticosteroid treatment are susceptible. Some fungal infections are short and self-limited while others are chronic.

Zoophilic infections (contracted from animals) usually provoke inflammatory reactions while anthropophilic infections (contracted from humans) usually do not.

Some fungal infections remain confined to one part of the body for a long time, for example, *Trichophyton rubrum* infection of the palm, or sole, while others spread extensively on the trunk and limbs, for example, *Trichophyton mentagrophytes*.

Some fungal infections, for example tinea pedis, provoke an ide reaction, a papulo-vesicular eruption on a site distant from the site of the actual infection.

Presentation of ringworm infections

Ringworm infections present in diverse forms in different parts of the body. The lesions may be annular, circinate, discoid or irregular dry scaly patches, inflamed exudative plaques, boggy swellings secondarily infected or hypertrophic or warty plaques. They are usually itchy.

A simple description of ringworm infections is according to anatomical sites: tinea capitis, tinea corporis, tinea manuum, tinea pedis, tinea unguium.

Tinea capitis (plates 9 and 10) Ringworm of the scalp commonest in children may present as patchy loss of scalp hair, the fungi having invaded the hair shaft and caused it to break. The affected scalp is usually dry and scaly but not inflamed.

Microsporum audouini (an anthropophilic fungus from humans) and *Microsporum canis* (a zoophilic fungus from pets) are the most common species.

Tinea capitis may become inflamed and secondarily infected by bacteria, producing a boggy painful lump (kerion: plate 10). Favus is a chronic infection covering most of the scalp with yellowish or brownish matted scabs and is caused by a *Trichophyton* or a *Microsporum*.

Tinea corporis Ringworm may invade any part of the non-hairy or hairy skin. The lesions may be dry and scaly or moist and inflamed depending on the dryness or moistness of the affected skin.

The most common presentation is the annular (ring-like) form with dry scaly irregular spreading edge which may be slightly raised or papular (plate 11).

The centre of the lesion is usually paler and smoother than the edge. The face, neck, trunk, arms and legs may be infected. Tinea corporis affecting specific sites are sometimes specifically named, for example, tinea barbae, tinea axillaris, tinea cruris.

Tinea cruris (figure 6.1) is common in hot humid climates especially when the standard of personal hygiene is low. It presents as an itchy spreading scaly eruption from the groins downwards to the thighs, backwards to the buttocks, inwards to the scrotum or vulva and upwards to the pubic region and lower abdomen. Neglected or badly treated tinea cruris can become secondarily infected or eczematised.

Trichophyton and *Microsporum* species are the commonest organisms causing tinea corporis. *Epidermophyton* is also among the causes of tinea cruris.

Tinea pedis Ringworm of the feet (sole, toe webs, sides of the toes, sides of the feet) may present as itchy dry, scaly, papular, vesicular,

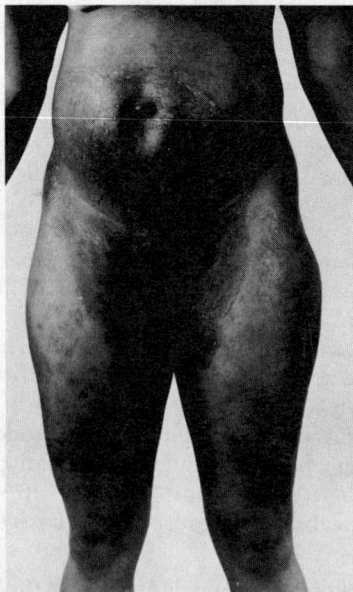

Figure 6.1   Tinea cruris: circinate scaly eruption with active edges involving groins and lower abdomen.

hypertrophic, fissured, inflamed, exudative, macerated or secondarily infected lesions. It is commoner in adults than in children.

Trichophyton rubrum and *Trichophyton mentagrophytes* are the commonest causes.

Tinea manuum Ringworm of the hands (palms, finger webs, sides of the fingers, sides of the hands) may present as itchy dry, scaly, papular, vesicular or hypertrophic lesions. It is less common than tinea pedis, and less common in children than in adults.

Trichophyton rubrum is the commonest cause.

Tinea unguium *(onychomycosis)* (figure 6.2)

Ringworm infection of the nails starts at the free edges of the nail and extends to involve most of the nail. The nails become discoloured and brittle. The nail bed is also invaded and fissuring, separation and crumbling of the nail plate result in ugly deformities of the nails. The infection may spread to other nails and toes or fingers. Toe nails are much more frequently infected than finger nails.

Tinea unguium is notoriously chronic and resistant to treatment.

Trichophyton and *Epidermophyton* are the commonest causes.

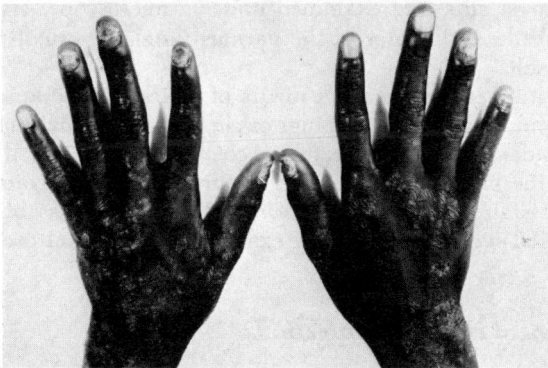

Figure 6.2   Tinea manuum and unguium: circinate lesions on dorsa of hands. Moth-eaten finger nails.

Diagnosis of ringworm (tinea) *infections*

This is based on:

(1) The clinical picture which in each case should be clearly differentiated from other conditions with which it may be confused. For example, tinea capitis may resemble alopecia

areata, pyoderma, seborrhoea capitis, trichotillomania or chronic discoid lupus erythematosus.

Tinea corporis may resemble pityriasis rosea, seborrhoeic eczema, nummular eczema, psoriasis or secondary syphilis.

Tinea cruris may resemble candidiasis, plain intertrigo of the groins, seborrhoeic eczema, flexural eczema or the bacterial infection, erythrasma.

Tinea pedis may resemble candidiasis, contact dermatitis, podopompholyx, keratoderma or plantar warts.

Tinea manuum may resemble candidiasis, contact dermatitis, cheiropompholyx or keratoderma.

Tinea unguium may resemble chronic paronychia, aspergillosis, nail dystrophy, psoriasis of the nails, nail biting, trauma, cosmetic staining of nails, contact dermatitis, nail discoloration by heavy metals or antibiotics.

(2) Wood's lamp often shows up fluorescence of various fungal lesions.

(3) Microscopic examination of skin scrapings, hair clippings, nail scrapings or clippings. The material is placed on a microscope slide, flooded with 40 per cent potassium hydroxide solution, warmed over a bunsen flame to digest the keratin, covered with a cover slip, and examined under a microscope. Hyphae or mycelia and spores of the various fungi are usually demonstrable.

(4) Culture in Sabouraud's media of scales, skin scrapings, hair clippings and nail scrapings or clippings will usually grow, in a few days to a few weeks, fungal colonies many of which produce in the media characteristic coloured stains, for example, the red stain of *Trichophyton rubrum*. Diagnosis is established by naked eye and microscopic examination of the culture growth.

Treatment of ringworm infections

Griseofulvin The antifungal antibiotic griseofulvin has revolutionised the treatment of various ringworm infections, but this effective and expensive drug is commonly misused

(1) When the diagnosis has not been made
(2) When the diagnosis is wrong
(3) When fungal infections which do not respond to griseofulvin, for example, tinea versicolor, candidiasis, are treated with it.

Griseofulvin acts by inhibiting the growth of fungi in skin, hair or nail after the drug has been absorbed in these tissues. It is effective against *Microsporum, Trichophyton,* and *Epidermophyton* infections.

It is given orally in tablet form (adults and children) or syrup (children who are unable to take tablets).

Dosage: microcrystalline tablets 250 mg q.i.d. (adults) or 250 mg b.d. (children).

Griseofulvin syrup 125 mg q.i.d. for children.

The duration of treatment depends partly on the site of the infection and partly on the chronicity. For early infections on the hairless skin or on the scalp, treatment for 4–6 weeks may be adequate. For chronic infections in the folds, hands, feet or nails, treatment may be necessary for 3–12 months. Tinea of the toe nails is the most stubborn to treat and reinfection may still occur even after treatment for over one year.

The side effects of griseofulvin include nausea, headache, urticaria and photoallergy.

Topical applications Numerous keratolytic agents had been used in the past, discarded and replaced. Most were only effective against small fungal infections with a short history.

Even the best available today are most effective when lesions are small, few in number and of recent origin.

(1) Whitfield's ointment, the old faithful compound ointment of benzoic acid made up of benzoic acid 5 per cent, salicylic acid 3 per cent, and soft paraffin 25 per cent in hydrophilic ointment.

It acts slowly shedding the horny layer with the mycelia and spores.
(2) Tolnaftate liquid, cream and powder. These preparations are cosmetically acceptable and reasonably effective.
(3) Haloprogin (Halotex) is about as good as tolnaftate.
(4) Clotrimazole (Canesten) is effective against ringworm infections, tinea versicolor and candidiasis.

All topical applications have to be used for at least a month after the lesion appears to have cleared.

6.4 **Candidiasis** (*moniliasis*) (figure 6.3 and plates 12 and 13)

Yeast-like fungi especially *Candida albicans* and *Candida tropicalis* can infect the mucous membrane of the mouth, anus and vagina and also the skin folds and nail folds. In debilitated children or adults, internal

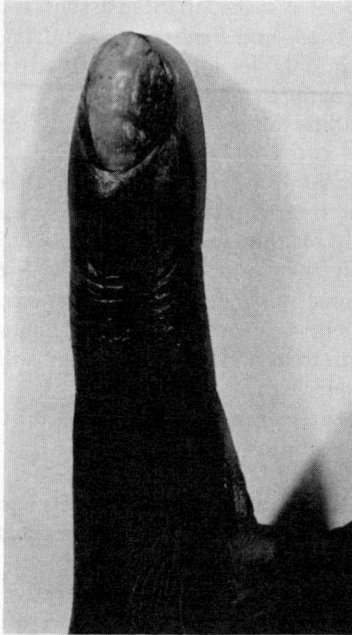

Figure 6.3   Chronic paronychia: bulbous nail fold and distortion of nail
plate.

organs such as the gut, urinary tract, bones, lungs, heart and brain
may be invaded. Following prolonged antibiotic or corticosteroid
treatment, superinfection with candida may also develop.

Thrush In infants, whitish, milky or greyish spots or sheets appear on
the tongue, lips, cheek mucosa and palate. The oral and vaginal
mucosa may also be affected. In immunocompromised or debilitated
patients, gastrointestinal and other visceral infection may follow and
can lead to death.

   Other conditions which predispose to systemic candidiasis include
thymus abnormalities, leukaemia, lymphoma and endocrine disorders.

Infection of skin folds In children and in fat, diabetic or debilitated
adults, pregnant women, dusky, reddish, raw or chalky eruptions
may develop in the large folds (axillae, breasts, groins, natal clefts,
flanks). Fissuring, eczematisation and secondary bacterial infection
may complicate the lesions.

Chronic paronychia The nail folds can be affected especially in people whose work involves frequent immersion of the hands or feet in water (housewives, doctors, nurses, dairy workers, bar tenders, washermen, bakers). The affected nail folds are swollen and tender and the nails may also be distorted or discoloured. Pus can often be expressed between the nail and the fold.

Interdigital candidiasis Inflammatory, erosive and fissuring lesions of the toe webs (commonly between the fourth and little toes) or finger webs (commonly between the middle and ring fingers). People engaged in wet work are most prone.

Vaginal candidiasis: Candida albicans may be nonpathogenic in the vagina in a number of normal women and more commonly in pregnancy. When it causes vaginitis, there may be pruritus, vaginal discharge and inflammation. The commonest differential diagnosis is vaginitis due to *Trichomonas vaginalis*.

Diagnosis of candidal infections

(1) History and clinical picture.
(2) Microscopic demonstration of *Candida* in swabs or scrapings from the mucosa, skin or nail fold.
(3) Culture of the material in Sabouraud's agar. Creamy or whitish colonies usually grow. From these candida can be demonstrated microscopically.

Treatment

For mucosal or superficial infections:

(1) Keeping the affected parts aired or dry.
(2) Gentian violet paint 1 per cent aqueous solution may clear mild infections.
(3) Mycostatin (nystatin) suspension or cream or ointment is more effective.
(4) Amphotericin B (Fungizone) cream or ointment.
(5) Clotrimazole (Canesten) solution, cream, ointment or vaginal tablets.
(6) Miconazole solution, cream or ointment.
(7) 5-Fluorocytosine solution.

For gastrointestinal tract infection:

> Mycostatin tablets 500,000 units q.i.d. for 1–2 weeks or Mycostatin suspension 500,000 units q.i.d. for 1–2 weeks. These are not absorbed and act locally on the gastrointestinal mucosa.

For systemic (visceral) infection causing gastroenteritis, septicaemia, endocarditis or meningitis, slow intravenous infusion of amphotericin B 0.25 mg–1 mg/kg body weight with 5 per cent glucose or dextrose.

Because of its toxicity to the gastrointestinal, renal, vascular and haemopoietic systems amphotericin B is used with care and only in the gravely ill. Clotrimazole and 5-fluorocytosine given systemically are effective but have the drawback of suppression of the haemopoietic system.

6.5   Deep fungal infections

Some fungi invade the deeper reaches of the skin as well as the underlying structures: fat, muscle, bone, joints and viscera.

6.6   Actinomycosis

Chronic granulomatous suppurative lesions on the face, neck, chest, abdomen or other sites.

Diagnosis

Demonstration of the organism (*Actinomyces israelii*) is made microscopically or on culture in swabs from discharging sinuses.

Treatment

Procaine penicillin in large doses. 1–5 million units daily until lesions clear up. In severe cases penicillin may have to be given intravenously. Tetracycline 1–2 g daily for 4–6 weeks or longer may also be effective. Surgical excision of infected tissue may be necessary.

6.7   Mycetoma *(madura foot)*

This is a localised chronic infection of the foot and leg caused by various species of fungi and actinomycetes.

The fungi or actinomycetes enter the body through broken skin and the infection spreads deeply. The leg and foot swell, nodules develop and extend to form granulomatous masses and secondary bacterial infection adds to the swelling, suppuration and disfigurement.

The nodules break down and discharge pus which tracks to the surface through sinuses. Underlying muscles, tendon and even bone become involved in the granulomatous process. The overlying skin becomes indurated and then verrucose.

The foot and leg are most commonly involved, but the buttocks, hands and other parts may occasionally be affected.

Diagnosis

This rests on the clinical picture, the demonstration of granules in swabs from discharging sinuses and the culture of the swabs to identify the causal fungi or actinomycetes.

Differential diagnosis

Conditions which may be confused with mycetoma include:

(1) Osteomyelitis. Microscopy of the pus will not reveal the granules, characteristic of mycetoma.
(2) Lymphoedema. This does not suppurate.
(3) Elephantiasis. This usually extends up the leg.
(4) Kaposi's sarcoma. The lesions are more nodular and haemorrhagic.
(5) Actinomycosis.

Treatment of mycetoma

There is no specific treatment for mycetoma but a combination of co-trimoxazole (Septrin) and dapsone 100 mg b.d. has been found useful in actinomycete infections. Griseofulvin 1 g daily has occasionally been helpful. Surgery may be resorted to when the foot is found useless.

6.8 **Histoplasmosis** (figures 6.4 and 6.5)

This is a subcutaneous, deep or visceral infection by various species of *Histoplasma*. *Histoplasma duboisii* the most common species found in Africa causes predominantly cutaneous and subcutaneous lesions.

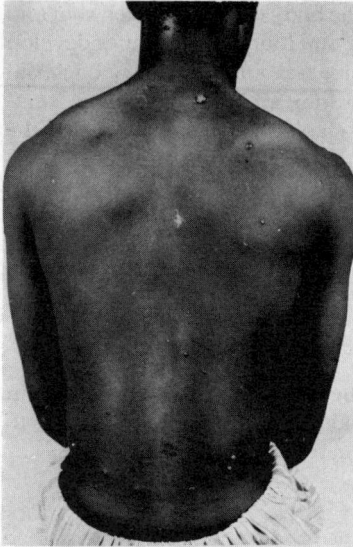

Figure 6.4   *(Left)* Histoplasmosis: deep-seated papules on trunk with umbilication and ulceration of older lesions.

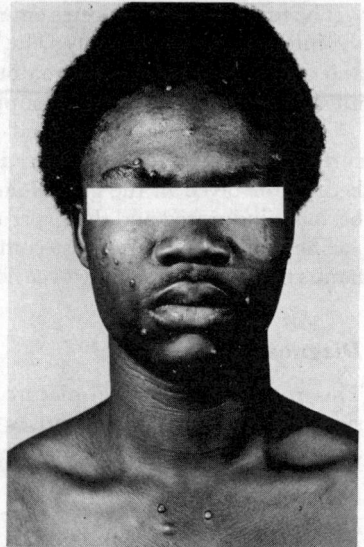

Figure 6.5   *(Right)* Histoplasmosis: umbilicated papules on face and chest.

The condition presents as cutaneous and subcutaneous papules and nodules which grow, umbilicate, suppurate and ulcerate. Lymph nodes may also be affected and in disseminated infections, the bones and lungs may become involved.

Infections with *Histoplasma capsulatum* usually cause pulmonary or disseminated histoplasmosis. They are commoner in the midwestern USA.

Diagnosis

(1) Isolation of the organisms in smears or biopsies.
(2) Culture of the organisms in Sabouraud's media.
(3) Histoplasma serology is usually positive but the histoplasmin skin test is not helpful in diagnosis.
(4) In systemic histoplasmosis, the organisms may be isolated from sputum, blood, or bone marrow.

Treatment of histoplasmosis

In spite of its toxicity, amphotericin B remains the drug of choice in a dose of 0.5–1 mg/kg body weight daily in 5 per cent glucose infusion.

6.9   Subcutaneous phycomycosis

This is a chronic deep fungal infection caused by a phycomycete. It develops insiduously and usually presents as a thick rubbery induration with a distinct edge deep under the skin. It is usually painless and feels somewhat like a thick slice of liver under the skin. The overlying skin is stretched but hyperpigmented. The thighs and buttocks are the common sites.

Diagnosis

This is based on the clinical picture, the histopathology and the isolation and culture of the fungi from biopsy specimens.

Treatment

The old drug potassium iodide solution given orally remains an effective and safe treatment. Dose 5–50 drops (in water or milk) daily in divided doses until the conditions clears up or improves. Griseofulvin, co-trimoxazole (Septrin) and amphotericin B intravenously have all proved useful in some cases.

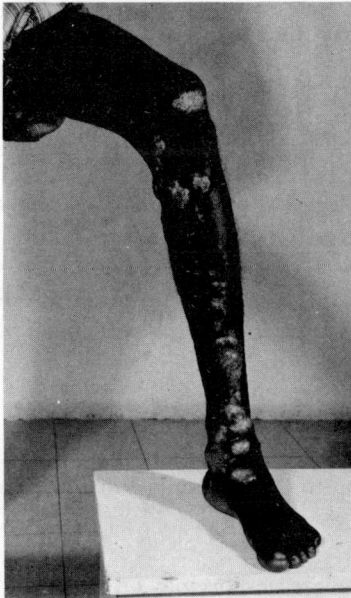

Figure 6.6   Chromomycosis: long-standing nodules, induration, ulceration and scarring (Courtesy: Dr J. U. Egere).

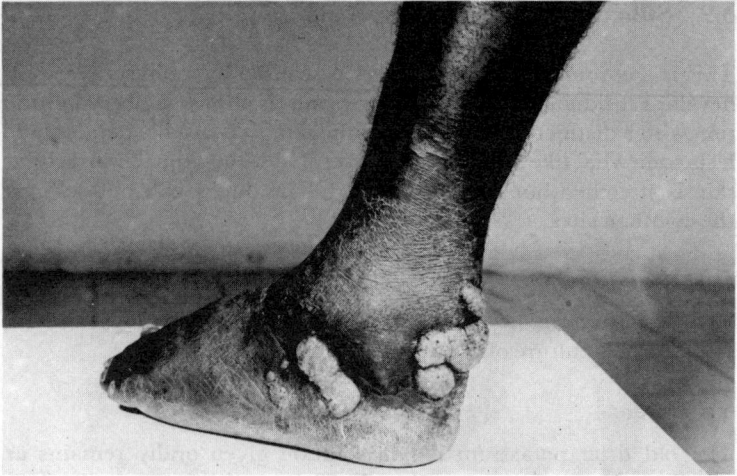

Figure 6.7   Chromomycosis: nodules around the ankle and oedema of the foot and ankle (Courtesy: Dr J. E. Egere).

6.10   **Chromomycosis** (figures 6.6 and 6.7)

This is a chronic deep fungal infection caused by various species of *Phialophora* and other pigmented fungi. It presents as warty nodules and plaques on the feet and legs. These may ulcerate and become secondarily infected with induration of the feet and legs. Lymphoedema of the feet and legs with verrucosity of the skin may develop.

Diagnosis

This is based on the clinical picture and the demonstration and culture of the fungi from biopsy specimens or scrapings from the hyperkeratotic plaques.

Differential diagnosis

Cutaneous tuberculosis (verrucose), Kaposi's sarcoma, syphilitic gummata and cutaneous leishmaniasis may present similar pictures.

Treatment

Excision of early solitary lesions may be curative.

Extensive lesions call for systemic treatment with intravenous amphotericin B or 5-fluorocytosine 6–8 g daily by mouth.

7   Viral Infections

These simple yet strange living organisms called viruses, each with a core of DNA (deoxyribonucleic acid) or RNA (ribonucleic acid) surrounded by a protein capsid, compel the living cells which they invade to manufacture more viral particles to the detriment of the cells.

Herpes simplex, a DNA virus disease, may present as mildly itchy grouped vesicles on a red or dusky base, lasting one or two weeks; as recurrent eruptions on the skin or mucosa; or as severe systemic viral infection. Antipyretic and antihistamines are helpful with mild infections while idoxuridine is effective against severe infections and gammaglobulin may be needed in systemic infections.

Varicella (chickenpox) and herpes zoster are caused by another DNA virus. Varicella, commoner in children, presents as a generalised eruption, while herpes zoster commoner in adults presents as localised bands or clusters of tense painful eruptions.

Other DNA virus diseases which cause severe illness include variola (smallpox), Kaposi's varicelliform eruption and infectious mononucleosis. DNA virus diseases affecting only the skin include molluscum contagiosum and warts of all types: common warts, plane warts, juvenile warts, plantar and palmar warts and ano-genital warts.

Two common RNA virus diseases both infectious fevers of childhood are rubeola (measles) and rubella (German measles). Measles presents as a generalised maculopapular eruption which may be complicated by keratoconjunctivitis, pneumonia, myocarditis and encephalitis.

Rubella presents as a short-lived eruption on the face and upper trunk. Its most dreaded complication is found in pregnant women. If the infection occurs in the first trimester, there is the risk of foetal malformations.

Viruses are extremely small intracellular parasites, much smaller than bacteria. Pathogenic viruses induce infected cells to manufacture viral components and synthesise new virus particles. They thus cause overgrowth and distortion or death of affected cells and produce characteristic clinical pictures.

Viruses cause a wide variety of skin diseases, from the trivial plane warts to the lethal smallpox, from the picturesque herpes zoster to the ugly condylomata acuminata.

7.1 **Warts** *(verrucae)*

These are benign tumours which begin as small papules or nodules on the skin or mucous membrane. They result from epithelial hyperplasia of the infected cells in which they grow, and usually appear after a variable incubation period of one to several months.

Warts are commoner in children than in adults. They are contagious and are spread by close personal contact. In children, warts are commonest on the hands, face and other exposed parts. The plane or juvenile warts have flat smooth surfaces slightly raised above the skin.

In adults warts are common on the feet and covered parts. The clinical variations depend on the dryness or moistness of the affected parts. They include common warts (verruca vulgaris) with rough or verrucose brownish or greyish surfaces, plane warts, juvenile warts, filiform warts and digitate warts which are thin and sessile, plantar warts and palmar warts which are painful and hyperkeratotic. Condylomata acuminata are soft, fleshy exuberant warts affecting the mucosa of the ano-genital region.

The course of warts is unpredictable. General or local immunity may account for the spontaneous regression of some warts.

Common warts *(verruca vulgaris)* (figure 7.1)

These are skin-coloured, dark brown, greyish or dark flat or rough-topped papules, nodules or plaques which may be asymptomatic or slightly itchy. The common sites are the hands, fingers, forearms and feet and lower legs.

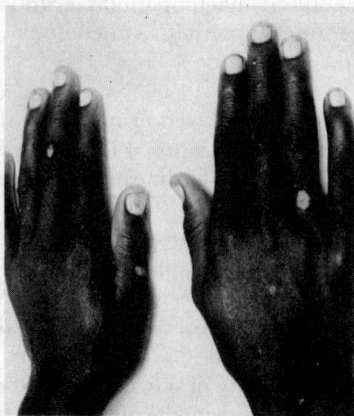

Figure 7.1   Verruca vulgaris (common warts) on dorsa of hands and fingers.

Plane, flat or juvenile warts *(verruca plana)*

These are small, flat, smooth skin coloured papules many of which may coalesce. Whether single, multiple or coalescent, they are only slightly raised above the level of the skin. A few indeed appear flush with the skin.

Plane warts are commonly found on the face and dorsum of hands and fingers. They are a disease of children and have a high rate of spontaneous resolution or regression.

Filiform and digitate warts *(verruca digitata)*

These are rapidly growing sessile skin-coloured or brownish projections which may be more cosmetically embarrassing than common warts. A single thread-like projection, filiform wart, usually appears near a muco-cutaneous junction, at the angle of the mouth, on the eyelid or elsewhere.

Multiple finger-like projections, digitate warts, have a broader base and the 'digits' are not as elongated as the solitary filiform wart.

Plantar warts *(verruca plantaris)*

The common form of plantar wart presents as one or a few hard painful and tender circumscribed calluses over the heels and balls of the feet. The centre of each wart is depressed and dark or pocked while the edge is raised and hyperkeratotic.

The rarer form (mosaic wart) appears as painful extensive plaques covering or almost covering the soles and pitted or honey-combed. Pressure and friction make plantar warts the most agonising of all warts. Plantar warts are usually chronic and defy many forms of treatment.

Palmar warts

These present as one or a few round or irregular hyperkeratotic nodules with depressed dark centres. They are painful because of the frequent friction of holding things in the hand. Palmar warts are far less common than plantar warts.

Ano-genital or genital warts *(verruca acuminata)* (figures 7.2 and 7.3)

These present as rapidly growing soft, moist dusky clusters on the muco-cutaneous junctions, mucosa or skin of these regions. They may be secondarily infected, foul-smelling and grow into ugly fungating or cauliflower-like masses. Many ano-genital warts but by no means all are sexually transmitted.

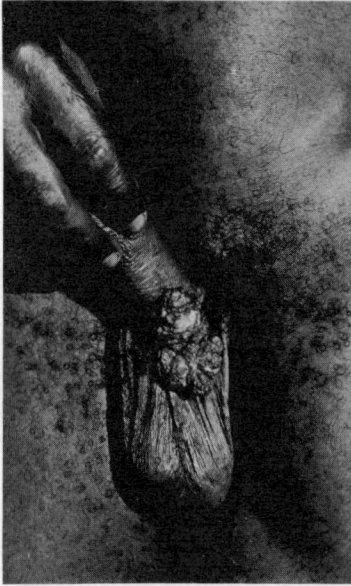

Figure 7.2   Genital warts involving the scrotum and penis.

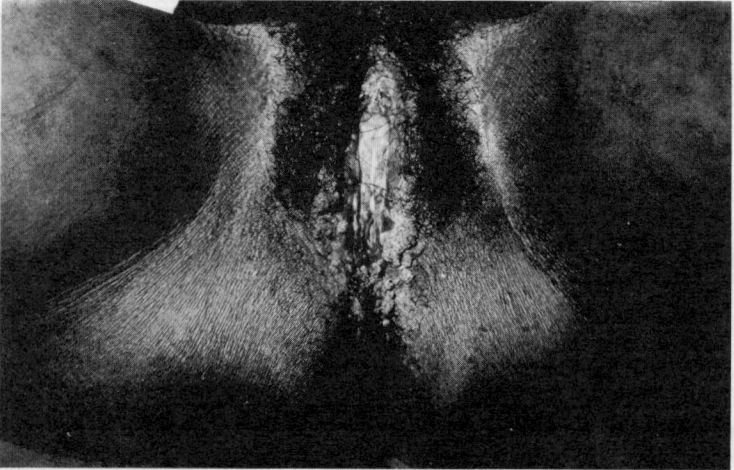

Figure 7.3   Genital warts involving the vulva.

Diagnosis of warts

This is based on the history and clinical appearance. Histological examination is seldom called for.

Conditions which may resemble warts are as varied as warts themselves: skin tags, molluscum contagiosum, lichen planus, seborrhoeic keratosis, actinic keratosis, cutaneous horn, plantar callosities, calluses, keratoderma, granuloma annulare, granuloma telangiectaticum, adenoma sebaceum, acne vulgaris, secondary syphilis, squamous cell epithelioma, keratotic and other naevi.

Treatment of warts

Spontaneous regression takes place in up to 60 per cent within 6–24 months. Only a proportion therefore require active treatment.

Local applications
  (1) Podophyllin resin, 25 per cent in alcohol. It is painful, and the normal skin should be protected with cotton wool or gauze. This is useful for ano-gential warts. 25 per cent of tincture of benzoin compound may be used in the same way as podophyllin.
  (2) Salicylic acid ointment 25 per cent with strapping. This is good for plane warts and verruca vulgaris.
  (3) 40 per cent salicylic acid adhesive plaster. This is also good for verruca vulgaris.
  (4) Freshly prepared liquor arsenicalis (Fowler's solution). This is good for ano-gential warts.
  (5) 10 per cent benzoyl peroxide cream applied twice daily for plane warts.

Chemical destruction Using phenol, formalin or nitric acid after curetting the warts. Verruca vulgaris is best suited for this method.

Cold surgery Freezing the warts with CO_2 snow or liquid nitrogen. This is used for verruca vulgaris and some plantar and palmar warts.

Diathermy Electrodesiccation and curettage under local anaesthetic. Digitate warts, plantar and palmar warts are best treated by this method. Filiform warts may be tied off with a black thread and allowed to drop off after a few days.

'Charming' of warts Making use of the knowledge that a proportion of simple warts regress spontaneously, a confident estimate of the time

of regression can be made, and the wart 'ordered' to disappear by then.

Plane warts, juvenile warts and verruca vulgaris in children are the ones best suited for this.

7.2   Herpes virus group

The common diseases in this group include herpes simplex (herpes febrilis), herpes zoster (shingles), and varicella (chickenpox). Herpes zoster and varicella are caused by the same DNA virus. In herpes zoster, the virus lies latent in the posterior root ganglia of spinal nerves until the infection is triggered off.

7.3   Herpes simplex

Crops of clear tense vesicles of variable sizes develop around the lips or other parts of the body when the body's resistance is lowered by fever, menstruation or other stressful situations.

Commonest sites – the muco-cutaneous junctions: lips, buccal mucosa, nose, eyes, ears, penis or vulva, buttocks.

The condition is usually subclinical or mild but may become complicated by secondary bacterial infection. In infants, severe mucosal infection may develop. In very severe cases viraemia may lead to meningo-encephalitis.

Treatment of herpes simplex

(1) Treatment of the underlying febrile illness.
(2) Relief of symptoms, for example, itching or pain.
(3) Antiseptic or antibiotic treatment of secondary bacterial infection.
(4) In cyclical herpes simplex in women, salicylates given a few days before the expected eruption may abort the eruption.
(5) Idoxuridine 1–5 per cent solution is most effective in herpetic keratitis but also useful in other herpetic infections.

7.4   Herpes zoster (figure 7.4 and plates 14 and 15)

This is an acute neurocutaneous infection by the same DNA virus that causes varicella. Prodromal symptoms of burning, pain or itching may precede the development of grouped tense vesicles on an erythematous or dusky base over the cutaneous distribution of one or more posterior roots of certain spinal nerves or of cranial nerves. The most commonly affected spinal nerves are the thoracic nerves particularly T_2-T_{10} and the most commonly affected cranial nerve is the fifth (trigeminal). Cervical, lumbar and sacral nerves are affected less frequently. Herpes zoster is more common in adults.

The affected area of the skin is hyperaesthetic. The band-like eruption is unilateral and markedly painful. The vesicles may break, become secondarily infected, scabbed, crusted or ulcerated leaving scars. Pain may persist in the involved area for months or years after healing. This post-herpetic neuralgia is more common in the elderly.

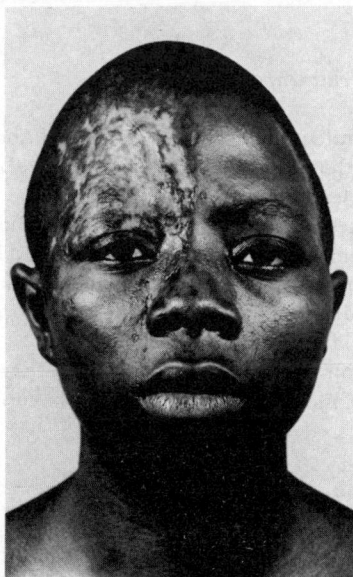

Figure 7.4   Herpes zoster: scarring over the cutaneous distribution of the ophthalmic division of the trigeminal nerve.

Complications of herpes zoster

These include keratitis in herpes zoster ophthalmicus, facial palsy in the Ramsay-Hunt syndrome, intractable post-herpetic neuralgia, herpes zoster encephalitis, and generalised herpes zoster especially when it is associated with leukaemia or lymphoma.

Treatment of herpes zoster

The objectives are to relieve pain and guard against post-herpetic neuralgia, to prevent, control or treat secondary bacterial infection and to manage the complications when they occur.

(1) Analgesics: these should be given in adequate doses to relieve pain.
(2) Calamine lotion with phenol or menthol.
(3) Antibiotics should be given systematically when secondary bacterial infection threatens or supervenes.
(4) Idoxuridine solution for the treatment of keratitis.
(5) Chlorpromazine (Largactil) 25–50 mg t.i.d. may be given for the management of post-herpetic neuralgia.

7.5   Varicella *(chickenpox)*

This is one of the infectious fevers of childhood and is caused by the same DNA virus that causes herpes zoster. Incubation period 1–3 weeks followed by fever and malaise.

Crops of clear, tense vesicles become widespread on the body, but are more profuse on the trunk than on the face and limbs.

The eruption is itchy. Secondary bacterial infection leads to ulceration and superficial scarring. The most infectious stage is from the day before the eruption for about one week.

In children, complications may include pneumonia, gastro-enteritis, nephritis, meningitis, and meningo-encephalitis.

Treatment

(1) Relief of itching.
(2) Antibiotics to guard against or control secondary bacterial infection.

7.6   Variola *(smallpox)*

Smallpox has been one of the scourges of man and occurred in epidemics killing many of its victims in areas where protection was inadequate. (The WHO recently announced that smallpox is now under control.)

Incubation period: 1–2 weeks.

Widespread papulo-vesicular eruption with umbilication leading to pustules and ulceration and leaving deep scars (pock marks). Lesions are more profuse on the face and limbs than on the trunk. Complications include secondary bacterial infection, toxic erythema, haemorrhagic lesions in skin and mucosa, pneumonia, eye complications leading to blindness and encephalitis.

The Medical Officer of Health must be notified if a case is diagnosed.

Treatment

(1) Isolation.
(2) Barrier nursing, maintenance of nutrition, antibiotic treatment.
(3) Prophylaxis: smallpox vaccination of whole populations.
(4) Administration of vaccinia immune globulin to susceptible smallpox contacts.

7.7 Measles

A common infectious fever of childhood. Incubation period 7–10 days. Diffuse maculo-papular eruption on a dusky reddish base associated with fever, upper respiratory tract infection, conjunctivitis and general constitutional upset. Complications include pneumonia, otitis media, dermatitis, meningitis, and encephalitis.

Treatment

(1) Relief of itching, fever, and muscle pains.
(2) Antibiotics to guard against secondary bacterial infection.
(3) Gamma-globulin injections to provide immediately usable antibodies.
(4) Prophylaxis: mass measles vaccination of all children.

7.8 Molluscum contagiosum (figure 7.5)

Molluscum contagiosum is a benign epithelial tumour of viral origin commoner in children than in adults. The virus of molluscum contagiosum is one of the largest viruses which affect man. Discrete glistening globular papules or nodules appear in crops. Large nodules show central umbilication. Lesions spread by auto-inoculation from the older lesions, and may be few or numerous. They may regress spontaneously or following secondary bacterial infection.

Treatment

(1) Curettage, touching the bleeding base with tincture of iodine or compound tincture of benzoin.
(2) Appropriate systemic antibiotics for secondary infected lesions.

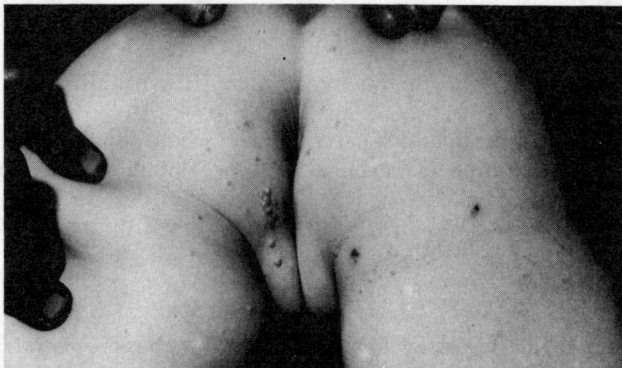

Figure 7.5   Molluscum contagiosum: globular papules on buttocks, inner thighs and vulva.

8 Eczema or Dermatitis

Attempts at exhaustive classification or description of eczema or dermatitis often confuse rather than clarify the subject.

The reaction pattern in the skin which may be called eczema or dermatitis is best classified simply according to the factors (exogenous, endogenous or atopic) which cause the reaction.

Exogenous dermatitis may be caused by toxic or caustic primary irritants (primary irritant dermatitis), by allergens (allergic contact dermatitis), or by light (photocontact dermatitis). Causes of exogenous dermatitis can be demonstrated by patch testing, and avoidance of such factors is a major step in treatment.

Atopic eczema due to inherited epidermal instability may present as infantile eczema usually starting on the face, flexures and trunk in the first six months; as atopic eczema starting in the flexures later in childhood; or as lichenfied atopic eczema affecting the flexures and trunk in adolescence or adult life. Atopic eczema may be associated with other manifestations of the atopic diathesis such as bronchial asthma, urticaria, hay fever and migraine.

Endogenous factors are responsible for the greasy scaly seborrhoeic eczema of the scalp and flexures common in infancy and childhood, for nummular or discoid eczema, for nutritional eczema, for dyshidrotic eczema of the hands and feet, for xerotic eczema, for neurotic eczema and for drug eruptions among others.

Management of endogenous and atopic eczema involves attention to environmental factors, the use of soothing applications, systemic medication, and the avoidance of irritants. Psychotherapy may be needed in some cases of atopic eczema.

Inadequate or wrong treatment of eczema or dermatitis may lead to generalised exfoliative dermatitis which can be life-threatening.

Inaccurate statements by earlier writers that darker skins were less liable to contact dermatitis, and that endogenous eczema was relatively rare in negroes have been disproved by current work.

Eczema or dermatitis is a common skin problem from which no region of the world is exempt. It now ranks next to infestations by animal parasites and bacterial infections among the commonest groups of skin diseases. It occurs in all ages and in all social classes.

The Greek word from which eczema was derived means 'to boil over'. This gives an accurate and dynamic ring to the mechanism by which epidermal cells become vesicular and progressively distended until they burst.

Eczema or dermatitis is a distinctive inflammatory reaction in the skin which is characterised in the early stages by any combination of the following primary lesions: erythema or duskiness, macules, papules, vesicles and bullae; and is usually accompanied by itching.

Eczema or dermatitis may be caused by exogenous factors (from outside the body) or endogenous factors (from inside) or by factors of epidermal instability which may be inherited or acquired.

The terms eczema and dermatitis are used synonymously. If any distinction is to be drawn, eczema may be used for reactions of endogenous or undetermined origin, while dermatitis may be used for reactions whose causes are exogenous and can be readily demonstrated by skin tests.

Broad classification is based on recognised aetiological background.

8.1   Exogenous dermatitis

This is caused by factors which reach the skin from outside the body, and are readily demonstrable.

Primary irritant dermatitis

An inflammatory reaction of the skin caused by strong acid, alkali, detergents, organic solvents or plant juices sufficiently concentrated to cause the reaction on anybody's skin. Primary irritant dermatitis tends to occur within 24 hours of contact with the substance. It is in the nature of a chemical burn and is more painful than itchy. The hands, face and other exposed parts are the usual sites. Contact with such primary irritants is usually accidental and at work.

Allergic contact dermatitis (figures 8.1 and 8.2 and plate 16)

An inflammatory reaction of the skin produced by a substance to which the skin had become sensitised usually by previous symptomless contact. It is a form of hypersensitivity, and takes days or weeks to develop. It is characterised by itching, redness or duskiness and papules or vesicles in the early stages. Common causes of allergic contact dermatitis include:

(1) Plant and vegetable products, for example, wood, wood products and wood dust.

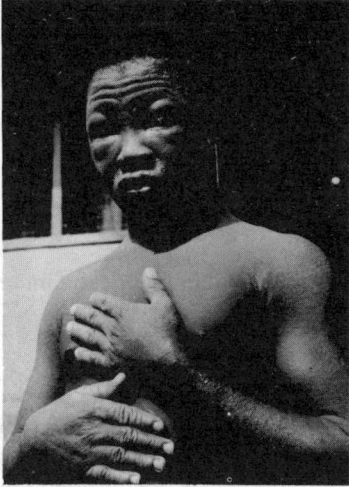

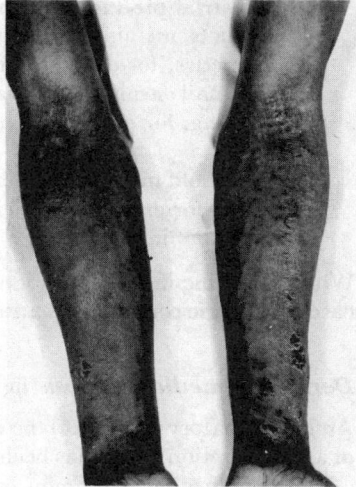

Figure 8.1   *(Left)* Allergic contact dermatitis due to hair dye.
Figure 8.2   *(Right)* Allergic contact dermatitis due to cement.

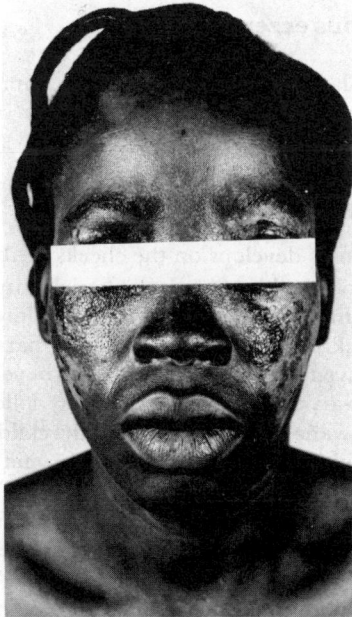

Figure 8.3   Dermatitis medicamentosa from medicated soap slush.

(2) Industrial products, for example, cement, rubber, petroleum products, metals, industrial fumes.
(3) Cosmetics, for example, hair dye, hair sprays and tonics, lip stick, nail varnish, deodorants.
(4) Clothing, for example, wool, synthetic materials, leather products.
(5) Household materials, for example, soap, detergents, polish.
(6) Drugs, for example, penicillin, streptomycin, sulphonamides, antihistamines.

With increasing industrialisation and sophistication, more and more cases of allergic contact dermatitis are being seen.

Dermatitis medicamentosa (figure 8.3 and plate 17)

An inflammatory reaction of the skin on the site and surrounding area of a skin eruption which has been overtreated or wrongly treated with a local application. Common causes of dermatitis medicamentosa include medicated soap, tincture of iodine, sulphur ointment, sulphonamide creams and antihistamine creams.

8.2   Endogenous eczema

This is caused by factors which reach the skin from inside the body, or by factors of epidermal instability which may be inherited or acquired.

Atopic eczema (figures 8.4 and 8.5 and plate 18)

Redness or duskiness develops on the cheeks at about the age of 3–6 months. This is followed by papules or vesicles and accompanied by itching. The condition may go on to affect the forehead and flexures especially the neck, elbows and knees. Other parts of the body may also become involved, or weeping and scaling develop in the subacute stage, and secondary bacterial infection may follow. The condition tends to wax and wane over the years and the child may grow out of it in early or late childhood. It may become chronic with thick scaling, lichenification and hyperpigmentation.

When atopic eczema starts in infancy, it is referred to as infantile eczema. Atopic eczema may, however, start in late childhood or even in adolescence.

Other atopic conditions with which atopic eczema may be associated either parallel with or appearing later in the same child

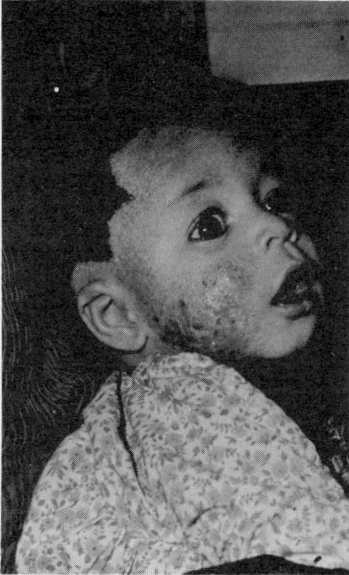

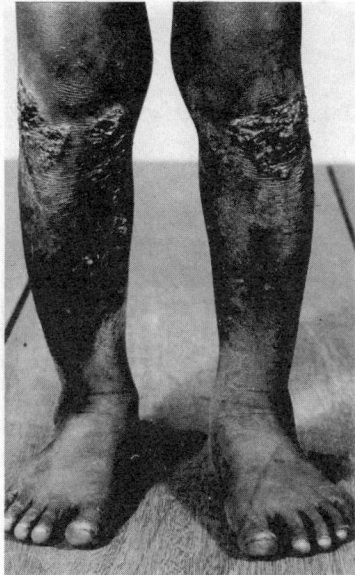

Figure 8.4   *(Left)* Infantile eczema: clusters of vesicles and scales on dusky
bases on cheeks and forehead.

Figure 8.5   *(Right)* Infantile eczema: exudative (weeping) and scaly plaques
on knees and lower legs.

include bronchial asthma, hay fever, urticaria and migraine. Children with atopic eczema may be sensitive, and should be treated with the minimum of fuss.

Seborrhoeic eczema (figure 8.6)

This is characterised by fine yellowish or brown greasy scales on the scalp, face, around the eyes, nose, mouth and ears, the axillae, neck, and the presternal and interscapular regions. These are the main sebum producing areas of the body. Other flexures and folds and the rest of the trunk may also become involved, and when severe may be dusky and exudative.

Seborrhoeic eczema is common in infancy, and then in late adolescence and in adult life.

Nummular or discoid eczema (figure 8.7)

This is characterised by itchy round or coin-shaped clusters of

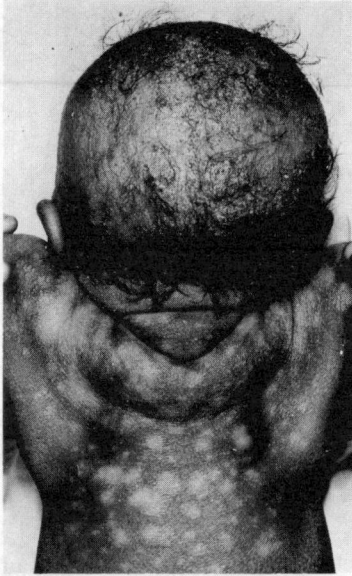

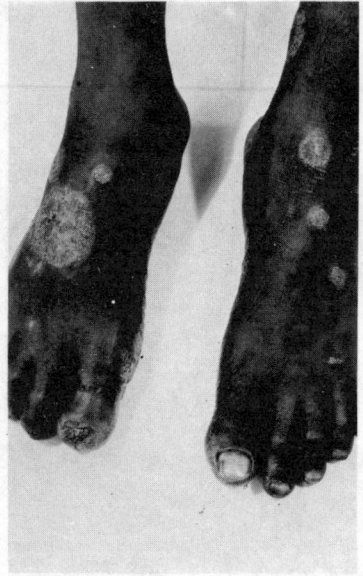

Figure 8.6   *(Left)* Seborrhoeic eczema: matted scales on scalp. Fine greasy scales on trunk and flexures.

Figure 8.7   *(Right)* Nummular eczema: coin-shaped scaly plaques on feet and lower legs.

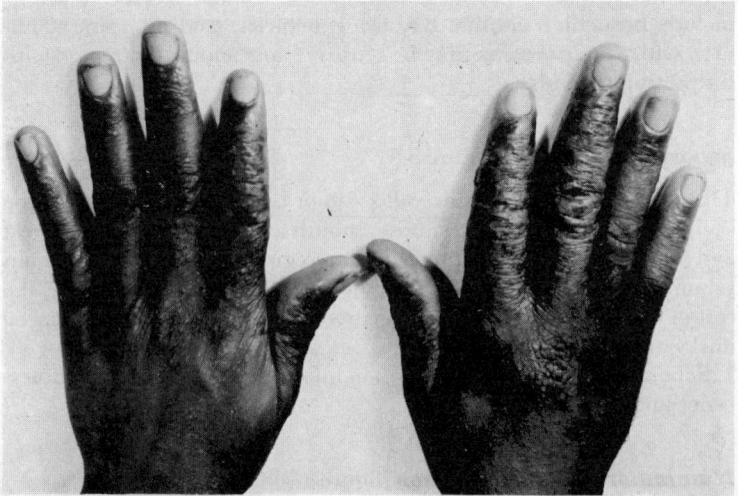

Figure 8.8   Eczema of the hands.

vesicles or scales on dusky backgrounds. Exudation, crusting, secondary infection or lichenification may follow. The extensor surfaces of the hands, the arms, legs and trunk are the usual sites, but other parts of the body may be involved.

Other examples of endogenous eczema (figures 8.8–8.12 and plate 19)

These include flexural eczema, flexural infective eczema, cheiropompholyx, podopompholyx, eczema of the hands and/or feet, eczema of the breasts, xerotic eczema, nutritional eczema, and neurodermatitis (lichen simplex chronicus).

8.3 **Generalised exfoliative dermatitis** (figures 8.13 and 8.14)

This, as the name implies, is a very extensive inflammatory reaction in the skin, characterised by profuse scaling all over the body.

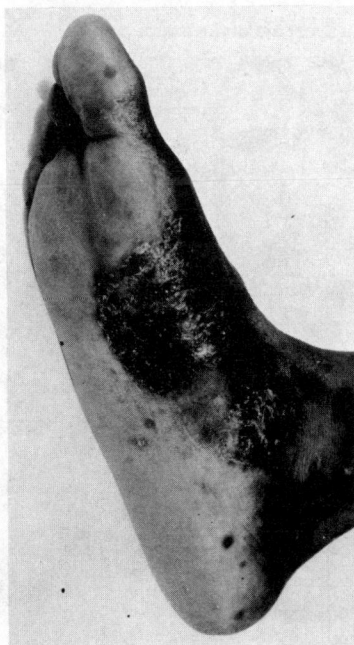

Figure 8.9   Eczema of the foot.

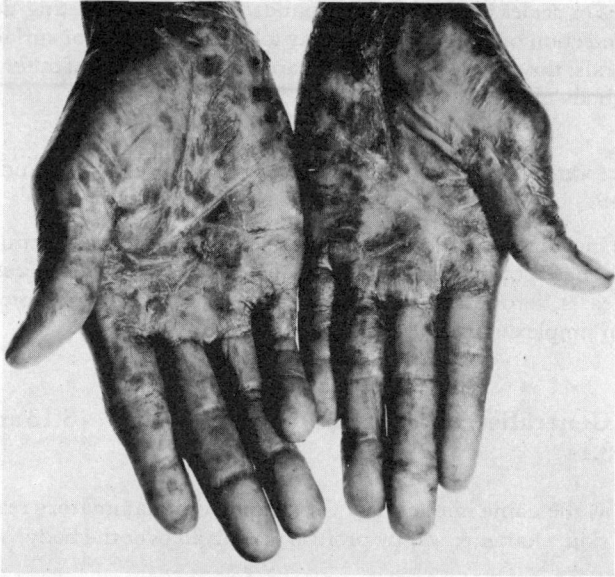

Figure 8.10   Chronic eczema of the hands.

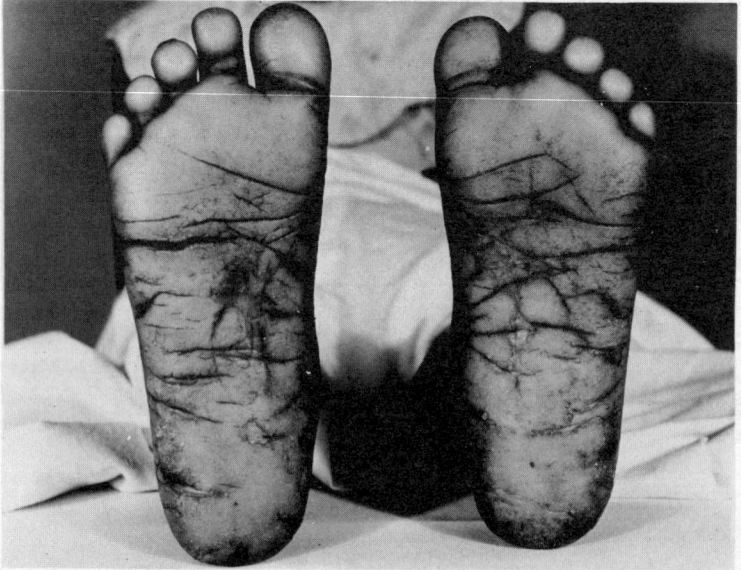

Figure 8.11   Chronic eczema of the feet with plantar hyperkeratosis and fissuring.

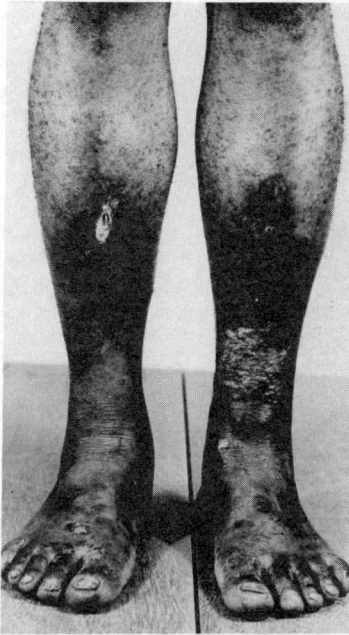

Figure 8.12   *(Left)* Chronic lichenified dermatitis.

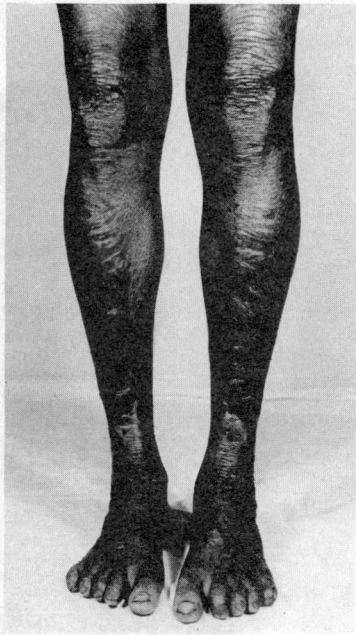

Figure 8.13   *(Right)* Generalised exfoliative dermatitis.

If there is generalised exudation, loss of fluid and protein and secondary bacterial infection can lead to general constitution upset and render the condition a threat to life. The condition can be a severe complication of exogenous dermatitis or of endogenous eczema, or it may develop on its own or as a reaction to drugs.

8.4   Stages of eczema or dermatitis

Many cases of eczema or dermatitis may pass through:

(1) Acute phase, with redness or duskiness, papules, vesicles or bullae and exudation or 'weeping'.
(2) Subacute phase, with secondary infection, scaling, fissuring and moderate thickening of the epidermis.
(3) Chronic phase, with scaling, lichenification, that is, pronounced thickening of the epidermis, and hyperpigmentation.

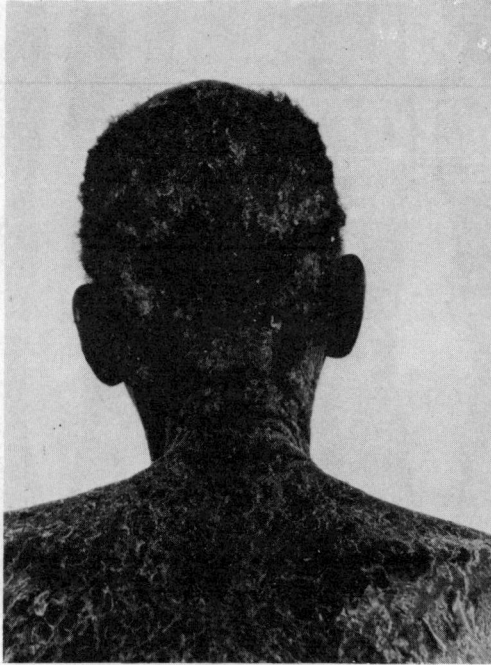

Figure 8.14   Generalised exfoliative dermatitis.

8.5   Histology of eczema or dermatitis

Eczema or dermatitis affects both the epidermis and the dermis, and all layers of the epidermis are thickened (acanthosis). The main histological changes seen from the horny layer inwards are:

(1) Increase in thickness of the horny layer (hyperkeratosis).
(2) Sponginess of the granular and prickle cell layers due to vesicle formation (spongiosis). These vesicles may break on the surface and 'weep' (exudation).
(3) Broadening and downward prolongation of the rete ridges.
(4) Vascular proliferation and perivascular round cell infiltration in the dermis.

8.6   Treatment of eczema or dermatitis

Success rests on finding the cause and removing it where possible;

relieving the symptoms; avoiding aggravating factors, for example, heat, repeated wetting, soaps, detergents, or friction; treating with topical applications and dealing with the complications if any.

First identify the cause (in exogenous dermatitis) and break the contact between the patient and the cause (primary irritant) or contact allergen.

Relief of symptoms (itching, burning or pain).

(1) Antihistamine drugs in common use include promethazine hydrochloride (Phenergan) 25 mg t.i.d., mepyramine maleate (Anthisan) 50 mg t.i.d. and chlorpheniramine maleate (Piriton) 4 mg t.i.d. These are available as syrup, tablet or injection.
(2) Sedatives, for example, barbiturates may be required in atopic eczema.
(3) Tranquilisers, for example, diazepam (Valium) 2–5 mg may be required in chronic lichenified eczema and neurodermatitis (lichen simplex chronicus).

Local treatment – different types of eczema or dermatitis call for different types of topical applications.

(1) In acute stage – wet dressings, for example, calamine lotion, corticosteroid lotion or spray. Betamethasone valerate, fluocinolone acetonide and flurandrenolone are among the best steroids.
(2) In subacute state – creams or ointment, for example, zinc cream; corticosteroid cream or ointment.
(3) In chronic stage – ointments or pastes, for example, zinc paste, coal tar paste, corticosteroid paste.
(4) In lichenified lesions and in neurodermatitis or lichen simplex chronicus – zinc paste, corticosteroid ointment with occlusive dressing, intralesional injection of corticosteroids.

Combined corticosteroid–antibiotic lotions, creams or ointments are available for eczema which is secondarily infected or is of infective origin.

Systemic antibiotics may be given for the control of secondary bacterial infection when this is present or is anticipated.

Systemic corticosteroids are indicated only in life-threatening generalised exfoliative dermatitis or other severe forms of dermatitis. Hydrocortisone hemisuccinate is given intravenously or in the infusion fluid until the patient can take prednisolone conveniently by mouth.

9 Papulosquamous Eruptions (Scaly Eruptions)

This group of diseases, characterised by papules as their main primary lesions and scales as their main secondary lesions, is presented in the order in which they occur in the tropical environment; pityriasis rosea, lichen planus, psoriasis. Standard works in the temperate regions would have the reverse order.

Pityriasis rosea presents with a dusky, oval, scaly eruption on the trunk, followed some days later by crops of smaller oval scaly eruptions on the trunk, neck, upper arms and thighs. The lesions usually fade within 6–12 weeks.

Lichen planus is more chronic, markedly itchy, presents as slaty-grey flat-topped papules or scaly plaques on the limbs and trunk, and is liable to become hypertrophic and disfiguring. Treatment is largely symptomatic and seldom dramatically successful.

Psoriasis presents as itchy thick dusky red lamellated scaly plaques on the scalp, extensor surfaces and friction area. It runs a very chronic course and seldom has the joint and nail involvement or occasional incapacitation found with psoriasis in the temperate region. Treatment is however, as difficult here as elsewhere, and this is testified by the host of topical and systemic treatments in use.

In this group of skin diseases the main feature is scale formation.

They are distinguished one from another partly by the length of the history and partly by the differing features of the scaling.

9.1 Pityriasis rosea (figure 9.1)

In this condition, a round or ovoid reddish or dusky rash (the herald patch) appears on the trunk or upper arm or thigh. This is followed a few days or about one week later by many (usually smaller) ovoid dusky scaly, macules distributed mainly over the 'shirt area' of the body, that is, trunk, neck, upper arms and thighs. Pityriasis rosea usually affects children or young adults, is slightly itchy, may last for 6–12 weeks and clear up spontaneously. It gives a mixed picture of an infection and an eczematous skin reaction. It is the commonest of the three scaly eruptions.

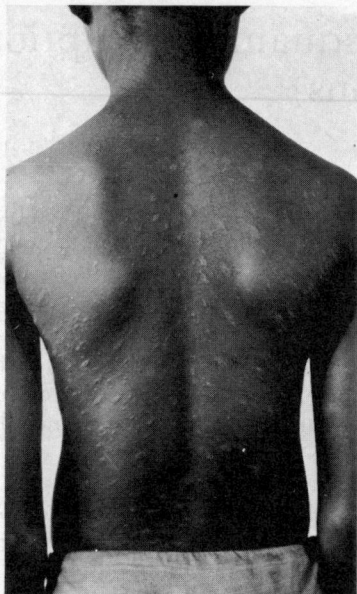

Figure 9.1   Pityriasis rosea: ovoid scaly macules on trunk with their long
axes parallel to the ribs.

Differential diagnosis

Pityriasis rosea may resemble tinea corporis, tinea versicolor, seborrhoeic eczema, psoriasis, and secondary syphilis.

Treatment

Because it runs this self-limited course, relief of itching with soothing
lotions or creams, for example, calamine lotion or corticosteroid
cream, and antihistamine syrup or tablets should be sufficient.

Wrong treatment with medicated soaps or irritant topical applications will usually produce a severe eczematous reaction.

9.2   Lichen planus (figure 9.2 and plates 20 and 21)

This eruption usually starts as small itchy papules on the wrists,
lower trunk or legs. These papules soon develop into shiny flat-topped
slaty-grey plaques, and lesions may spread to involve many parts of
the body. Lesions on the shin and ankles tend to become hyper-

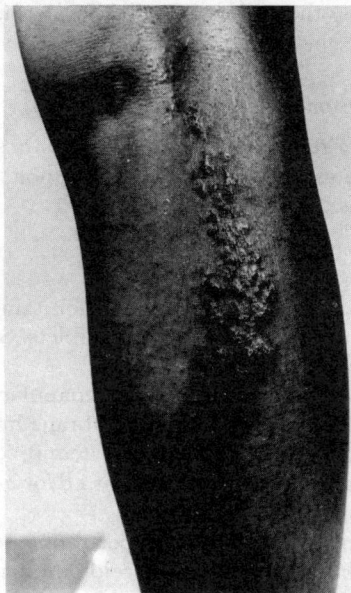

Figure 9.2   Lichen striatus: column of grey keratotic papules and plaques
streaking from the ankle across the calf to the thigh.

trophic. Whitish, creamy or greyish lesions inside the mouth (cheeks,
tongue or lips) are common and may last longer than the skin lesions.
Occasionally the nails are distorted.

The condition may last for many months and as it subsides, the
lesions leave dark macules which may take some years to clear up.
Lichen planus shows the Koebner phenomenon. This means that
lesions may develop on sites of scars or over scratch marks on the skin.

Lichen planus is more itchy, more disfiguring to the skin, more
upsetting to the patient and more difficult to treat than pityriasis
rosea. Lesions may become bullous, florid or generalised with marked
increase in itching, and some constitutional upset. Lichen planus may
be triggered off by stress. It is more common in adults than in
children. The cause is unknown but psychogenic and autoimmune
factors have been postulated.

Histology

The main features are hyperkeratosis, hypergranulosis, acanthosis,
saw-toothed appearance of the rete ridges, and a band of lymphocytic

infiltration hugging the undersurface of the dermo-epidermal junction and the upper one third of the dermis.

Differential diagnosis

Lichen planus may resemble psoriasis, secondary syphilis, lichenoid drug eruption, for example, mepacrine eruption, other drug eruptions, lichen simplex chronicus.

Treatment

(1) Relief of itching with calamine lotion, zinc cream, corticosteroid creams, and antihistamine tablets. Sedation with barbiturates may be necessary.
(2) In acute **widespread** or generalised papular or bullous lichen planus, and in severe mucous membrane involvement or nail destruction, a short course of systemic corticosteroids, for example, Tab. prednisolone 10 mg t.i.d for 2–3 weeks tailed off thereafter.
(3) Management of the chronic hypertrophic lesions with tar or zinc paste dressing or corticosteroid ointment under occlusive dressing or with intra-lesional injection of corticosteroids.

9.3   Psoriasis (figures 9.3 and 9.4)

This condition, rare in the tropics, is characterised by dusky thick lamellated scales on the scalp, elbows, knees, the extensor surfaces of the limbs generally, and the trunk and waist. The lesions may have geometrical patterns and the edges are sharply demarcated.

When fully developed, the plaques of scales are thicker, more defined and larger than in lichen planus and the distribution should distinguish it from lichen planus. It tends to itch less than lichen planus.

Other striking clinical differences include more frequent involvement of the nails, palms and soles in psoriasis, involvement of the joints in some cases of psoriasis, normal colour of healed areas of psoriasis.

Some cases are flexural in distribution while others present with generalised small papules (guttate psoriasis).

Psoriasis runs a chronic course of many years, punctuated by periods of complete or incomplete clearing of scales either spontaneously or as a result of treatment. It is the least common of the three scaly eruptions being described.

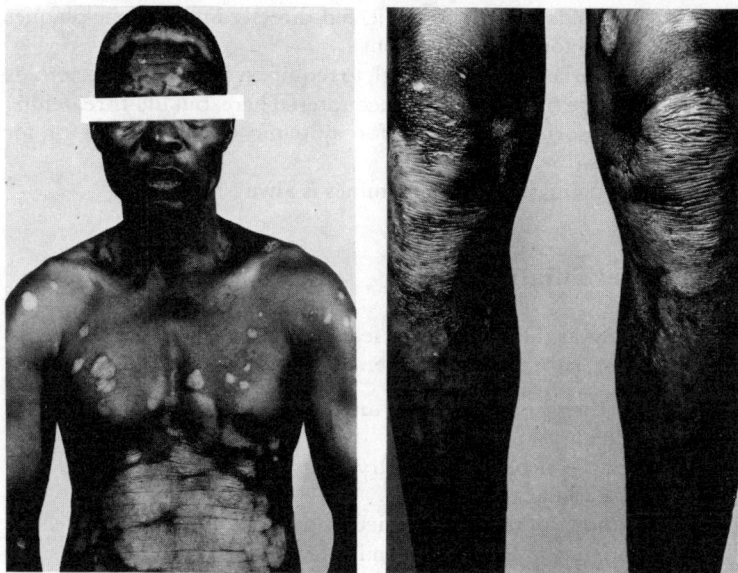

Figure 9.3   *(Left)* Psoriasis: thick scaly plaques on scalp, trunk and extensor surfaces of legs and arms.

Figure 9.4   *(Right)* Psoriasis: thick scaly plaques on knees and shins.

Psoriasis may start in childhood, and patches of psoriasis may persist into old age and the patient may die from some other disease or from old age. There is often a family history of psoriasis.

Treatment

This has never been easy and this is testified by the host of local and systemic treatments which had been tried over the years with varying success and more frequent failure.

Acceptable topical applications currently considered useful include

(1) After a tar bath and removal of scales weak dithranol ointment is applied.
(2) One per cent coal tar paste.
(3) Anthralin in zinc oxide and salicylic acid paste.
(4) Corticosteroid ointment with or without cellophane or plastic paper wrap.

Corticosteroids can also be injected directly into chronic plaques which resist all topical applications.

Cases of psoriasis severe enough to require systemic corticosteroids or methotrexate have not been encountered here, but life-threatening generalised psoriasis will call for systemic corticosteroids or for methotrexate.

Relief of itching with antihistamines is always helpful.

9.4   **Differential diagnosis**

With scaliness as the outstanding feature of these three papulosquamous eruptions, care should be taken to distinguish them from

(1) Seborrhoeic eczema. Finer and more greasy scaling in the scalp and flexures.
(2) Tinea versicolor. Finer dry scaly sheets in presternal and interscapular regions.
(3) Eczema or dermatitis. Vesicular or exudative phases may have a tendency to become secondarily infected.
(4) Secondary syphilis. Lesions are more papular than scaly, involve the palms and soles, and serological tests for syphilis are positive.

10 Allergic Reactions and Bullous Eruptions

Altered tissue reaction to substances with which the body had previously come into contact may be viewed as a protective reaction aimed at stopping further absorption of the offending substances. The reaction may be mild as in simple urticaria, moderate as in erythema multiforme or severe as in anaphylaxis.

Patterns of skin eruptions associated with such allergic reactions include urticaria, angio-oedema, papular urticaria, purpura, erythema multiforme, Stevens–Johnson syndrome, erythema nodosum, and granuloma annulare. Some may be traced to allergens in food or drugs, some to underlying viral or bacterial infections and others to physical factors. The treatment is usually dictated by the underlying cause discovered.

The bullous eruptions considered here are probably due to auto-immune reactions. They include dermatitis herpetiformis, herpes gestationis, pemphigus of the various types (p. vulgaris, p. vegetans and p. foliaceus) and pemphigoid. Dermatitis herpetiformis responds to sulpha derivatives (diaminodiphenyl sulphone and sulphapyridine) while pemphigus calls for systemic corticosteroid therapy.

Allergy is an altered reaction of tissues to substances with which they had previously come in contact. Some allergic reactions are beneficial, for example, antibody reactions to infections and vaccines; while others are harmful, for example, anaphylactic reactions and auto-immune reactions.

Some of these allergic reactions are bullous and need to be distinguished from bullous eruptions of auto-immune or other aetiology.

10.1 Urticaria

This is a common disorder characterised by the sudden or gradual appearance of itchy usually transient raised weals of variable shapes and sizes on any part of the skin or mucosa. The weals are pale, normal coloured or dusky, and pitted like orange skin.

Weals may vary from pin-head sized ones to those many centimetres across. They may be round, ovoid, annular or irregular, sometimes assuming picturesque geographical patterns.

Weals may last a few minutes, hours, days or weeks. Some cases persist and become chronic. Severity varies from the mildest form to anaphylaxis with peripheral vascular collapse. With peripheral vascular collapse, death may supervene unless prompt and adequate resuscitation is available.

Mechanism of production of weals

Mast cells in the dermis are important in the production of weals. The release of histamine from mast cells may be triggered off by antigens, immunoglobulins or complement.

The skin swelling is due to localised tissue oedema following cutaneous vasodilation in response to released histamine or other vaso-active chemicals, for example, bradykinin, kallikrein, acetylcholine and prostaglandins. There is usually no tissue destruction and when the weal subsides there is little or no sign that any lesion had been there.

Common causes of urticaria

Multiple factors are often involved, some allergic, others non-allergic or mixed.

Allergic urticaria, usually acute is due to allergens reaching the body through the mouth, through the skin or through mucosal membranes. In immediate urticarial reactions, scratch skin tests with the offending substance are usually positive.

(1) Through the mouth: foods of plant or animal origin, alcoholic and non-alcoholic drinks, drugs, (aspirin, codeine, oral penicillin) microorganisms and intestinal parasites.

(2) Through the skin: insect, fish and other animal stings, injections, for example, penicillin, anti-tetanus serum, plant and animal bristles, bacteria and other microorganisms and animal parasites, for example, filariasis.

(3) By inhalation: insecticides, plant sprays, deodorants, and chemical fumes.

The onset of allergic urticaria may be delayed for days and scratch skin tests may be negative.

Chronic urticaria may be associated with infections, systemic diseases, reticulosis, auto-immune diseases, neoplasms, and may not be demonstrably allergic. Some allergic reactions may become chronic.

Physical factors such as heat, cold, or pressure may provoke urticaria. Heat urticaria may follow exposure to heat or severe exercise. Cold urticaria may follow contact with cold air, ice block or cold metal. Physical pressure such as the edge of a table or chair or the sling of a bag or a belt or corset may produce a weal.

In dermographism, stroking the skin with a pen will raise a weal in a few minutes (figure 10.1).

Familial, hormonal and psychogenic factors may also play a part in heat urticaria, solar urticaria, cold urticaria, dermographism and other forms of urticaria.

In many cases of urticaria, no cause can be found by methods of investigation now available.

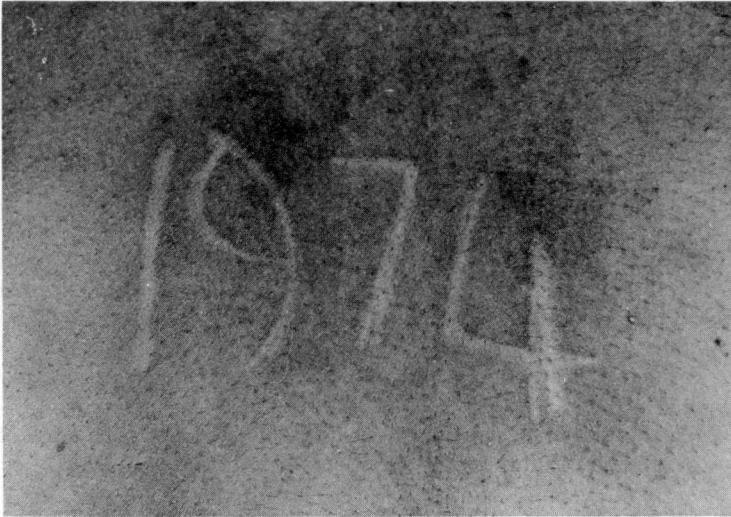

Figure 10.1   Urticaria: dermographism demonstrated.

Differential diagnosis

Conditions which may be confused with urticaria include insect stings or bites, erythema multiforme, localised lymphoedema, localised myxoedema and renal disease.

Treatment of urticaria

The most important step is to try to identify the cause and eliminate or avoid it. Recovery usually follows this. Antihistamines orally or by injection usually control urticarial eruption.

In severe or extensive lesions, adrenaline 1 ml of 1/1000 solution should be given subcutaneously, slowly. This may be repeated after 15–20 minutes if necessary. In anaphylactic reactions or angio-oedema, intravenous hydrocortisone may be life-saving.

10.2 **Angio-oedema**

In this severe variant of urticaria, there is sudden or gradual swelling of the mucosa and subcutaneous tissues. The lips, nose, eyes, tongue, and larynx swell moderately or grotesquely and breathing and swallowing become very difficult. Bronchospasm and gastrointestinal upset (nausea, vomiting, abdominal cramps) may follow. The cause may be food, drugs or other agents as in simple urticaria.

Treatment must be prompt and adequate if distress is to be relieved and the threat to life removed. Antihistamines by injection and adrenaline are called for, and even hydrocortisone may be required.

10.3 **Papular urticaria**

This disorder presents as a recurrent or chronic eruption of itchy, dusky papules or clusters of papules and pustules on the exposed parts or covered parts. An early urticarial element is replaced by inflammatory papules which become secondarily infected.

Papular urticaria is seen commonly in children, and is due mainly to insect bites (bedbugs, fleas, mites, sand-flies) the urticarial eruption and subsequent secondary bacterial infection often being out of proportion to the number or severity of the insect bites.

Treatment

Control of the home, nursery or school environment by the use of insecticides will reduce the incidence of insect bites.

Antihistamine syrup or tablets and calamine lotion or other soothing creams will allay the itching. Secondarily infected cases should be treated with the appropriate antibiotics.

10.4 **Purpura**

Purpura is the stippling of the skin or mucous membranes by red blood cells which escape through the capillaries as a result of capillary damage, thrombocytopenia or other factors. When the purpuric spots are small, they are known as petechiae and when large, as ecchymoses.

Purpura may be produced by infections, drugs or systemic diseases which cause platelet disorders, capillary damage or coagulation disorders.

Treatment of purpura is by treatment, correction or avoidance of the underlying factors. Drugs which can produce thrombocytopenia, for example, quinidine, quinine, barbiturates, sulphonamides, chlorothiazide, digitoxin and oxytetracycline should be used with care.

10.5   Erythema multiforme (plate 22)

This is an acute eruption with a diversity of lesions in various combinations: erythema, dusky or dark macules, papules, vesicles, iris lesions, bullae, discs, rings, purpura and urticaria.

Erythema multiforme may be associated with fever and constitutional upset. It may be cyclical or recurrent.

Its causes are as diverse as its lesions, but three of its common and readily demonstrable causes are viral infections, bacterial infections and drugs (sulphonamides, barbiturates, salicylates, phenolphthalein, penicillin, dapsone).

The common sites of the lesions of erythema multiforme are the face, especially around the mouth, hands and feet, ano-genital region, forearms and knees.

Mucosal membranes may be involved in some cases. In toxic erythema multiforme (Stevens–Johnson syndrome) there is extensive erosion of the mucosa of the eyes, mouth, throat and external genitalia resulting in secondary bacterial infection and severe constitutional disturbance and fluid and electrolyte loss.

Treatment of erythema multiforme

(1) In the mild localised bullous and papular or urticarial type, relief of itching or burning with antihistamines.
(2) If the disorder is due to a drug, this should be withdrawn.
(3) If it is due to infection, this should be treated.
(4) Secondary bacterial infection of lesions of erythema multiforme should be treated or prevented.
(5) In toxic erythema multiforme, systemic corticosteroids may be used to combat the condition, fluid and electrolyte loss should be corrected, and secondary bacterial infection should be treated.

10.6   **Erythema nodosum**

This is a nodular dusky or erythematous eruption usually seen on the extensor surface of the lower legs or on the arms, thighs or other parts of the body. The nodules are usually tender and may be acute or run a prolonged course. When the nodules heal, they tend to leave hyper-pigmented macules.

Common causes of erythema nodosum are tuberculosis, leprosy (erythema nodosum leprosum), fungal infections, bacterial infections (for example, streptococcal infections), and drugs (for example, sulphonamides).

Treatment of erythema nodosum depends on the cause which should be treated, eliminated or avoided.

10.7   **Granuloma annulare** (figure 10.2)

This is slowly developing nodular ringed or button-shaped eruption seen mainly in children and young adults.

It presents as skin-coloured or dusky or pale taut palpable rings or circinate plaques with raised or beaded edges and flat normally pigmented centres. The common sites are the dorsa of the hands and fingers, wrists, ankles, feet, forearms and legs.

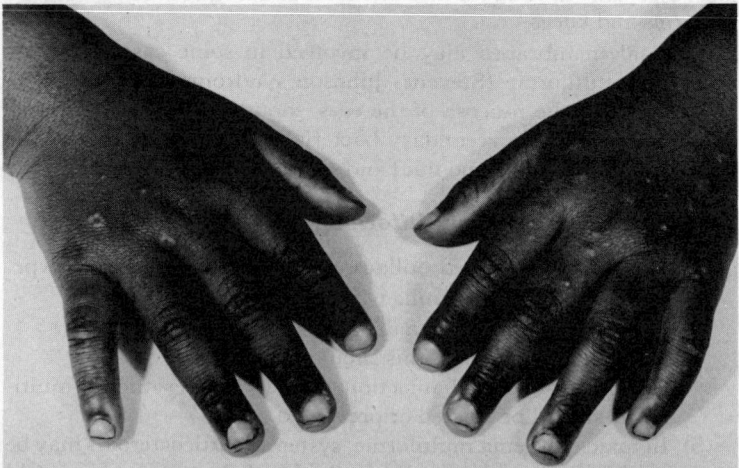

Figure 10.2   Granuloma annulare: numerous ring-like or button-shaped swellings on the dorsa of the hands and fingers.

Granuloma annulare is painless and non-itchy. The lesions may be solitary, localised and few in number, or widespread on the body. They may last from a few months to a few years and when they resolve spontaneously, the lesions leave no scars. Recurrences may however occur. A papular form scattered and non-annular may be seen occasionally.

The cause of granuloma annulare is unknown. Some lesions have been associated with tuberculin tests, insect bites, or other forms of scarification.

In adults necrobiosis lipoidica diabeticorum may be confused with granuloma annulare especially histologically.

Treatment

Many lesions resolve spontaneously though slowly and require no treatment. Intra-lesional injection of triamcinolone or other corticosteroids helps the resolution of lesions. Biopsy of granuloma annulare may be followed by resolution of the rest of the lesion.

10.8 Dermatitis herpetiformis (*Duhring's disease*)

This is a rare skin eruption characterised by recurrent crops of dusky bullae with an admixture of vesicles, papules and urticarial weals. The lesions are symmetrical, and itching is usually intense. Ingestion of iodides usually causes a flare-up.

The extensor surfaces of the trunk and limbs are usually more severely affected. Scratching leads to the breaking of the vesicles and bullae with secondary bacterial infection. Healed lesions leave hyperpigmented macules or pigmented superficial scars. Dermatitis herpetiformis runs a long course with alternating periods of exacerbation and remission.

A variant of the disease, herpes gestationis may occur in pregnancy. When it does, it may subside before childbirth or persist after it with exacerbations related to the menstrual periods.

Diagnosis

This is based on a history of recurrent pruritic vesicles and bullae responding poorly to treatment. The bullae are deep-seated, usually subepidermal, with eosinophils the predominant cells within the bullae.

Differential diagnosis

The bullae of scabies and impetigo contagiosum are more superficial and fragile.

The bullae of erythema multiforme last much shorter periods.

The bullae of pemphigus are usually associated with mucosal lesions.

The bullae of epidermolysis bullosa start in childhood, are more prominent over pressure areas, and leave thin atrophic scars and sometimes dystrophy of the fingers and toes.

Treatment

Dapsone 100–200 mg daily usually produces remissions.

Sulphapyridine 0.5 g t.i.d. is also useful but has more side effects than dapsone. Antihistamines are given for the control of itching. Corticosteroids help to control the itching, and allow the use of lower doses of other drugs. Corticosteroids are more effective than dapsone and sulphapyridine in the treatment of herpes gestationis.

10.9   Pemphigus

This is a chronic and debilitating bullous disorder which is commoner in middle age and old age. It is thought to be an auto-immune disease. Autolysis of epidermal cells occurs with development of intra-epidermal bullae. Pemphigus presents in three main forms.

Pemphigus vulgaris In this condition, the acantholysis occurs in the deeper parts of the epidermis and the bullae are suprabasal. The bullae break and the raw tender surfaces become crusted over. Healing is slow and new bullae erupt on new or old sites. Oral or other mucosal erosions precede or accompany the skin lesions.

The prognosis is poor and mortality is high from electrolyte imbalance, protein depletion, fluid loss, infection and septicaemia unless adequate treatment is available.

Pemphigus vegetans In this variant, the bullae are also suprabasal. These also break and vegetations or thick granulations develop at the edges as more bullae erupt.

The course is longer and the prognosis slightly better than in pemphigus vulgaris.

Pemphigus foliaceous In this variant, the bullae are more superficial.

The lesions may resemble exfoliative dermatitis with vesicles, crusts and scales. It occurs in younger people.

The course is usually prolonged but the prognosis is much better than in the other variants.

Treatment of pemphigus

Systemic corticosteroids have altered the previously hopeless prognosis of most forms of pemphigus. They have to be given in large doses to control the condition.

Prednisolone 100–150 mg daily in divided doses should be given until the eruption of fresh bullae is controlled. The dose is then gradually reduced to a maintenance dose.

Because of the high dosage of corticosteroids and the immediate dangers of gastric irritation or haemorrhage, the tablets should be given after meals and a watchful eye kept on gastric symptoms.

10.10 Pemphigoid

This condition of the elderly resembles pemphigus but is less severe. The bullae may be preceded by urticarial and eczematous eruptions. The bullae are subepidermal rather than suprabasal.

Corticosteroids are also useful and should be given in high doses with the same care about side effects.

11 Drug Eruptions

Drugs taken for the cure of a disease or for the relief of symptoms may produce undesired side or toxic reactions in the body. These reactions may be due to overdosage, intolerance, hypersensitivity or idiosyncrasy. They may be mild, moderate, severe or even fatal. Any system in the body may be involved: cutaneous, gastrointestinal, haemopoietic, reticulo-endothelial, cardiovascular, respiratory, hepatic, urinogenital or nervous. Drugs may also alter the microflora or affect the skin's response to actinic radiation.

Drug eruptions (cutaneous drug reactions) may present with various combinations of primary and/or secondary lesions: erythema, macule, papule, nodule, vesicle, bulla, weal or urticaria, pustule, exudate, crust, scab, scale, erosion, ulcer, scar, keloid, cyst, lichenification, plaque, hypopigmentation, hyperpigmentation. The drug eruption may also mimic specific skin disorders, for example, eczema or dermatitis, pyoderma, pityriasis rosea, lichen planus, acne vulgaris, psoriasis and skin tumours.

The difficulty in correctly diagnosing drug eruptions lies in the fact that while each primary or secondary skin lesion can be produced by a large number of drugs, each drug can also produce a wide range of skin lesions. A common drug like aspirin can produce urticaria, purpura, erythema multiforme and fixed eruption, and urticaria can be produced by aspirin, penicillin, anti-tetanus serum, sulphonamides, antimalarials, and barbiturates to name only a few.

Management of drug eruptions rests on correct identification of the offending drug and its avoidance. In severe life-threatening reactions, for example, anaphylaxis, heroic measures such as systemic corticosteroid therapy and tracheostomy with positive pressure respiration may be required.

11.1   Drugs in common use and their common eruptions

Examination of the most commonly used drugs and the various eruptions they commonly produce would appear the simplest starting point:

Aspirin: urticaria, purpura, erythema multiforme, fixed eruption, pruritus.

Penicillin: urticaria, vesicles, bullae, exfoliative dermatitis, anaphylactic shock, Stevens–Johnson syndrome. Penicillin topical applications are also photosensitisers.

Sulphonamides: erythema, erythema multiforme, erythema nodosum, toxic epidermal necrolysis, fixed drug eruption, urticaria, exfoliative dermatitis. Sulphonamide topical applications are also photosensitisers.

Streptomycin: eczema, exfoliate dermatitis, erythema multiforme.

Antimalarials: pruritus, urticaria, pigmentation, fixed drug eruption, exfoliative dermatitis, lichenoid eruption.

Antihistamines: Photosensitivity is caused by promethazine hydrochloride (Phenergan). Urticaria, purpura and fixed drug eruption may be caused by other antihistamines.

Diaminodiphenyl sulphone (dapsone): fixed drug eruption.

Clofazamine (Lamprene): skin pigmentation.

Progestogens (oral contraceptives): hyperpigmentation, chloasma, acne, urticaria, erythema nodosum, alopecia, hirsutism.

Broad-spectrum antibiotics: tetracycline may stain the teeth in children and the nails in children or adults. It can also produce fixed drug eruption. Its prolonged administration may alter the gastrointestinal bacterial flora and lead to candidiasis.

Isoniazid: urticaria, purpura, acneiform papules.

Diphenylhydantion: gingival hypertrophy, erythema, fixed drug eruption, exfoliative dermatitis.

Phenolphthalein: fixed drug eruption, urticaria, bullae.

Barbiturates: urticaria, erythema, fixed drug eruption, dermatitis.

Phenothiazines: skin pigmentation.

Antitetanus serum: urticaria, anaphylactic reaction.

Corticosteroids: acneiform papules.

Management of drug eruptions

When a correct diagnosis has been made on the basis of a good history, the offending drug should be withdrawn unless the risk from the disease against which it was being given is greater than the risk from the drug reaction.

Antihistamines may be given to control pruritus.

Corticosteroids may be given in severe drug reactions.

11.2   Fixed drug eruption (figures 11.1 and 11.2 and plate 23)

This presents in the early stages as itchy erythematous or dusky macules which soon become vesicular or bullous. They later rupture,

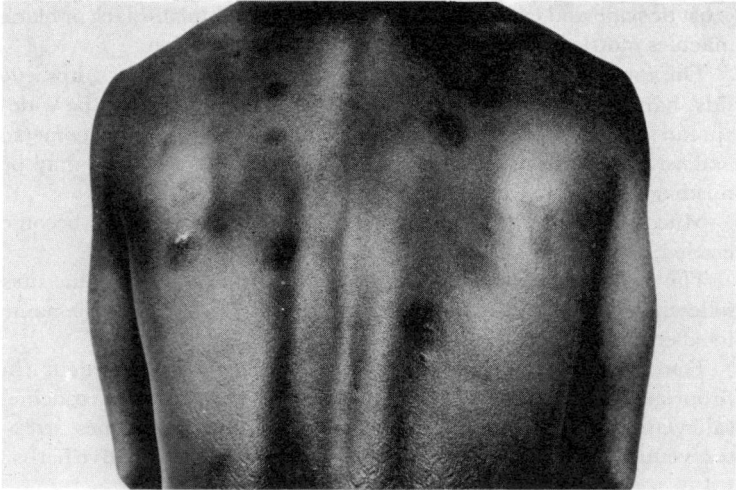

Figure 11.1 Fixed drug eruption: circinate bluish-black macules on the trunk.

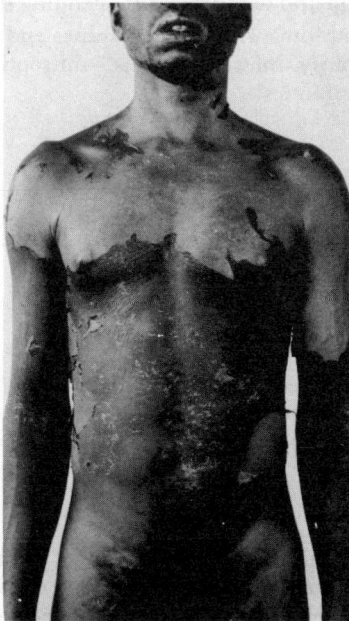

Figure 11.2 Fixed drug eruption: severe reaction with extensive bullae breaking to leave raw areas.

crust or scale and eventually heal, leaving dark, bluish-black or black macules mottled with perifollicular hyperpigmentation.

The common sites for fixed drug eruption include the face, lips, eye lids, hands, external genitalia. The lesions may, however, be widespread on the face, neck, trunk and limbs. They may become so extensive that the islands of normal skin appear pale and may be misdiagnosed as leprosy or vitiligo.

Mucosal lesions (lips, tongue, external genitalia) may become eroded.

The eruption has the striking tendency to recur on the same sites following subsequent exposure to the causal drugs, hence the name fixed eruption.

The drugs commonly implicated include phenolphthalein (in proprietary laxatives), sulphonamides, antimalarials, codeine, salicylates, dapsone, chlortetracycline and other tetracyclines, streptomycin, barbiturates, phenylbutazone, arsenicals and native herbs.

Treatment of fixed drug eruption

(1) Identification and withdrawal of offending drug.
(2) Relief of symptoms with antihistamines and soothing lotions.
(3) For secondarily infected lesions, antiseptic applications or systemic antibiotics.

11.3 Penicillin reactions

This great antibiotic which is very much in use, and its use very much abused, causes many allergic skin reactions.

Immediate reaction including anaphylaxis

This may occur immediately after injection, with manifestations including generalised pruritus, flushing, fear, weakness, dysponea, angio-oedema, bronchospasm, vascular collapse and shock.

Delayed reaction

This may occur within 1–3 weeks and may manifest as urticaria, fever, joint pains, angio-oedema, lymphadenopathy, proteinuria. Other possible reactions include erythema, eczema, exfoliation, purpura, erythema multiforme, and fixed drug eruption.

Treatment of severe penicillin reaction

(1) Adrenaline 1 ml of 1/1000 solution subcutaneously slowly. This may be repeated in 15–20 minutes if necessary.
(2) Hydrocortisone hemisuccinate 100 mg I.V. or dexamethasone 4 mg I.V. or I.M.
(3) Antihistamines, for example, diphenhydramine hydrochloride 10 mg I.V. or chlorpheniramine maleate 10 mg I.M.
(4) In bronchospasm, 250 mg of aminophylline I.V.
(5) Oxygen inhalation and artificial respiration. Tracheostomy may be needed in extreme emergencies.
(6) If penicillinase is at hand, its administration may lessen the severity.

11.4 Anti-tetanus serum reactions

These may also be immediate or delayed.

Immediate reaction, including anaphylaxis

There may be sudden development of pruritus, urticaria, angio-oedema, bronchospasm and vascular collapse.

Delayed reaction

This may occur after one or more weeks. The skin and mucosal reactions develop more slowly but can become as severe as the immediate reaction and include anaphylaxis.

Treatment

As in penicillin reaction above.

12 Skin Disorders Associated with Malnutrition

When inadequate intake, absorption, or utilisation of nutrients, including vitamins, results in clinical vitamin deficiency disease, many tissues may show stigmata of such deficiency. The skin and its appendages and mucous membranes often bear the outward visible signs of a systemic deficiency.

The bulk of skin diseases associated with malnutrition show protein and vitamin B lack. This is in consonance with the low content of protein and vitamin B in many staple diets in the tropics and subtropics.

Kwashiorkor (severe protein calorie malnutrition) hits the skin in various ways while pellagra and phrynoderma show distinctive cutaneous eruptions and aneurine and riboflavine deficiencies affect the skin and other organs.

Prompt and adequate treatment of vitamin deficiency diseases with the appropriate vitamins usually improves the clinical disorders. Improvement in socio-economic conditions is needed to prevent these diseases of underdevelopment and undernutrition.

Skin diseases associated with malnutrition usually result from deficiency of many rather than of single food factors or vitamins. The clinical pictures may be clear-cut as in severe kwashiorkor and in pellagra or may be indistinct as in hypovitaminosis – B.

12.1 Vitamin A deficiency

Vitamin A deficiency is usually associated with deficiency of other vitamins. It seldom manifests as an isolated feature.

The accepted features include dryness of the skin, follicular keratosis, xerophthalmia and impaired night vision.

Treatment

Vitamin A by mouth and a diet rich in vitamin A, for example, milk and eggs, and carotene-rich vegetables should be given.

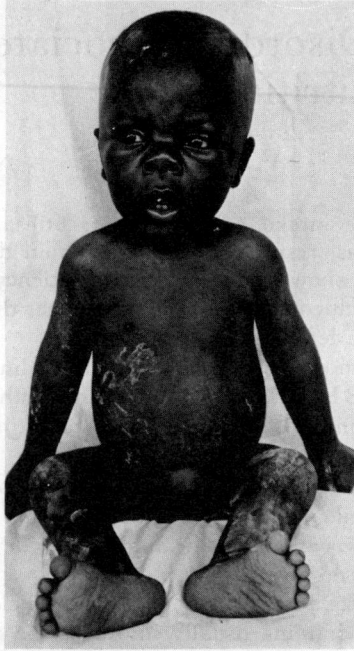

Figure 12.1   Kwashiorkor with skin desquamation (Courtesy: Dr Winifred Kaine).

12.2   **Kwashiorkor** (figure 12.1)

In this condition of severe protein calorie malnutrition seen most commonly in young children, muscle wasting, oedema, fatty infiltration of the liver and retarded skeletal and mental development are the main features. The skin changes include:

(1) Generalised loss of pigment. Part of this appearance is due to stretching of the skin from oedema.
(2) Duskiness leading to hyperpigmentation in the flexures, pressure points, face, hands and feet and other areas, giving a pellagroid picture.
(3) Scaling and peeling of the hyperpigmented skin leaving raw areas.
(4) Blistering and rupture of the hyperpigmented areas, leaving raw skin which is really infected and may ulcerate.
(5) Patches of dry cracked skin on face, trunk and limbs ('crazy paving').

Mucous membrane changes include glossitis, magenta tongue, angular cheilitis, rhinitis, conjunctivitis, and vulvovaginitis.

The normally beautiful black curly hair loses its texture, its lustre and its fullness, and becomes thinned out and straight. It undergoes colour changes – brown, yellowish, ginger, reddish, or even blonde.

Treatment

(1) Dietary treatment with reconstituted dried skimmed milk, increasing the strength as improvement is obtained.
(2) Multivitamin supplements and iron should be given.
(3) Correction of electrolyte imbalance by giving Darrow's solution and glucose orally.
(4) Investigation and prompt treatment of intercurrent infection and/or worm infestation.
(5) Public health education.
(6) Improving the socio-economic standard of the community.

12.3 **Phrynoderma** *(follicular hyperkeratosis)* (figure 12.2 and plate 24)

This condition is characterised by grouped spinous or papular eruptions distributed mainly over the extensor surfaces and areas of

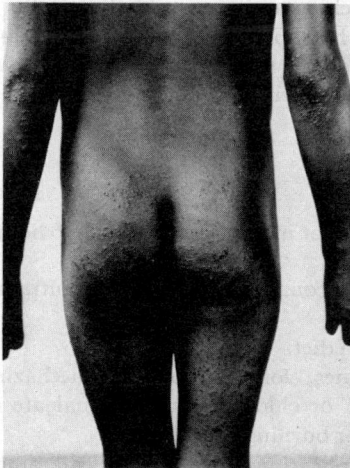

Figure 12.2 Phrynoderma (follicular hyperkeratosis): spinous papular eruption on extensor surfaces and pressure areas.

friction – elbows, ulnar borders of the forearms, shoulders and scapular regions, buttocks, thighs, and knees. There is generalised roughening of the skin and the affected areas feel decidedly spinous to touch. Phrynoderma is due mainly to vitamin B deficiency.

Treatment

   (1) Vitamin B complex tablets or syrup b.d.
   (2) Vitamin B complex injection 1–2 ml I.M. on alternate days for 4–8 weeks.
   (3) Improved diet to include animal and vegetable proteins.

12.4   **Pellagra** *(nicotinic acid deficiency)* (figures 12.3–12.5 and plate 25)

The striking feature is the involvement of the exposed parts of the skin – the back and sides of the neck, the dorsa of the hands, wrists, the feet and shins. The affected skin first becomes dusky, and may become oedematous, vesicular or bullous, the area desquamating and leaving sharply demarcated hyperpigmented areas. Glossitis and angular cheilitis may also be seen. Exacerbations of skin erythema and other lesions sometimes follow exposure to sunlight. Symptoms may include burning, itching or pain, and diarrhoea. The dementia to complete the text book picture of 'dermatitis–diarrhoea–dementia' is seldom seen, but there may be apathy. Pellagra is due to deficiency of nicotinic acid and/or tryptophan in the diet.

Treatment

   (1) Nicotinic acid or nicotinamide 100 mg 6 hourly until condition improves.
   (2) Vitamin B complex orally and intramuscularly as in phrynoderma.
   (3) High protein diet.
   (4) Antihistamines, for example, promethazine hydrochloride (Phenergan) or chlorpheniramine maleate (Piriton) to allay the itching or burning sensation.
   (5) Soothing applications, for example, calamine lotion.
   (6) Control of gastrointestinal symptoms if present, for example, diarrhoea, with antidiarrhoeal mixtures or tablets.

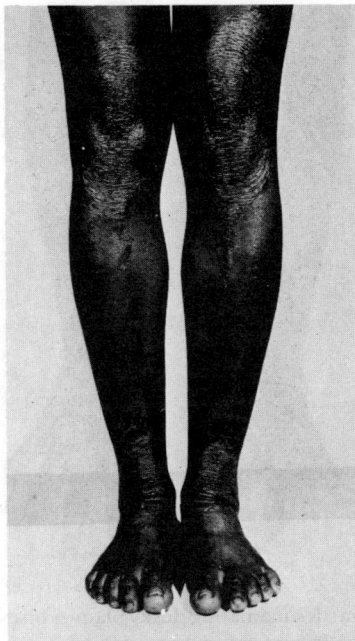

Figure 12.3   Pellagra: flaky hyperpigmented plaques on legs.

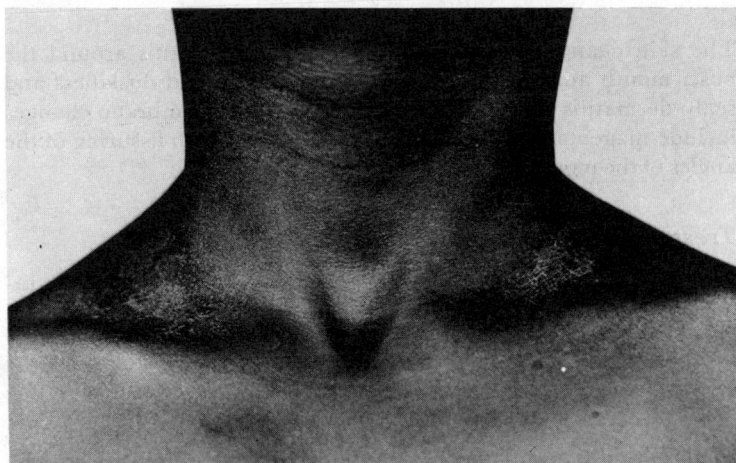

Figure 12.4   Pellagra: flaky hyperpigmentation on sides of the neck.

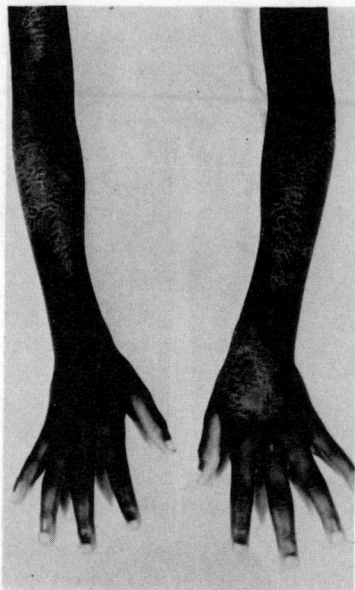

Figure 12.5   Pellagra: desquamating dusky plaques on extensor surfaces of the arms, forearms and dorsa of hands.

12.5   **Riboflavine deficiency**

The skin changes include dyssebacia (oily dermatitis around the nose, mouth and ears), fissuring of the mouth, and duskiness and scaly dermatitis of the scrotum. Oral mucosal membrane changes include magenta tongue, cheilitis and perleche with fissuring of the angles of the mouth.

Treatment

Riboflavine 5 mg t.i.d. orally. Riboflavine may be given by intra-muscular injection. The dietary errors should be corrected.

12.6   **Aneurine** *(thiamine deficiency)*

In this condition, cutaneous eruptions are not prominent but the paraesthesia, numbness, foot drop, wrist drop and oedema of the

hands and feet may be associated with a flaky dermatitis and devital-
isation of the skin with ulceration.

The more prominent features of aneurine deficiency (beriberi) are
usually neurological: paraesthesia, numbness, foot drop and wrist
drop. There may also be myocarditis, oedema of the face, hands and
feet and gastrointestinal disturbances.

12.7 **Hypovitaminosis – B** (figure 12.6)

Moderate degrees of vitamin B deficiency not amounting to one of the
more specific syndromes may result in dryness of the skin with
patches of hypopigmentation in the extensor surfaces and pressure
points, diffuse palmo-plantar hyperkeratosis and magenta tongue.

Treatment

Vitamin B complex orally or by intramuscular injection.

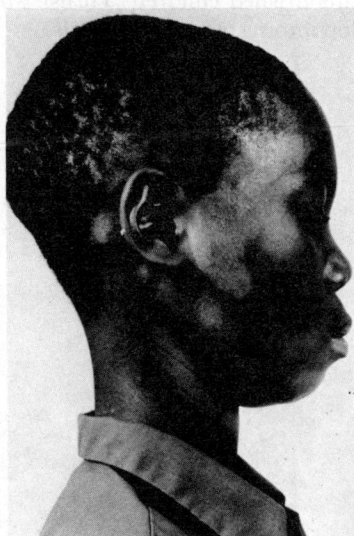

Figure 12.6   Hypovitaminosis – B: hypopigmented fine scaly patches on the
face and extensor surfaces of the arms.

12.8   **Vitamin C deficiency** *(scurvy)*

Features of vitamin C deficiency may be seen on the skin as haematomas or smaller perifollicular haemorrhages; in the mouth as gingivitis and bleeding gums; or on the hairs as broken hairs or spinous processes resembling phrynoderma.

Other features include anemia, defective wound healing, irritability and depression.

Treatment

Ascorbic acid 100 mg t.i.d should be given and the diet enriched with fresh fruits and vegetables.

12.9   **Effect of malnutrition on other skin diseases**

In malnourished patients, especially children, bacterial infections, viral infections and fungal infections tend to become more severe.

Impetigo contagiosum may develop into ecthyma. Herpes simplex may develop into a fatal viraemia. Post-measles dermatitis becomes more severe in malnourished children. Thrush and cutaneous candidiasis may develop into systemic candidiasis.

13 Disorders of Pigmentation

The right amount of the pigment melanin is essential for good health. Too little or too much is usually embarrassing. Too little or none at all increases the proneness to actinic radiation and the train of skin damage ending up with skin cancer.

Vitligo or leucoderma, hypopigmentation, hyperpigmentation and hypermelanosis may be associated with various systemic diseases. Management of the underlying diseases counts more than local treatment of the pigmentary disorders.

The ravages of time and the elements on the skin of albinos make them very prone to skin cancer and calls for the continuing care of the skin of albinos from very early life, using sunscreens, protective clothing and career counselling.

The colour of the skin is determined by a number of factors: the brown pigment (melanin) in epidermal cells, the yellowness of plasma in living epidermal and dermal cells, the redness of the dermal blood vessels, and the thickness of the horny layer of the epidermis.

Melanin is produced in the skin by the melanocyte which contains many melanosomes. Premelanosomes, the precursors of melanosomes possess tyrosinase activity. This enzyme tyrosinase catalyses the amino acid tyrosine to dihydroxyphenylalanine (dopa), and dopa is then oxidised in stages to melanin.

Melanin is also produced by the same mechanism in the hair bulb adjacent to the hair papilla.

Melanin granules are transferred from the melanocyte through its dendritic processes to adjacent basal cells or to the cortex and medulla of the hair shaft. Ultraviolet light stimulates increased melanin formation, increased oxidation and darkening of melanin granules and increased upward migration of melanin granules within epidermal cells.

Melanin production is under the influence of the melanocyte-stimulating hormones (MSH) of the intermediate lobe of the pituitary gland.

Physiological variations in melanocyte activity in melanin production results in individual and racial differences in degree of melanin pigmentation, but the number of melanocytes does not vary with race.

Disorders of pigmentation often genetically based but sometimes acquired may result from:

(1) Biochemical abnormalities involving the tyrosine-tyrosinase (amino acid-enzyme) system.
(2) Changes in structure or location of the melanocytes.
(3) Under-stimulation or overstimulation of the melanocytes by melanocyte-stimulating hormones.
(4) Defective melanin acceptance by diseased, damaged or abnormal epidermal or hair cells.
(5) Toxic or side-effects of drugs. Disorders of pigmentation may be a decrease or an increase. Either way, the patient may be worried, and those who see him may become suspicious.

13.1 Vitiligo *('white skin')* (figures 13.1 and 13.2 and plate 26)

This is a disorder of pigmentation in which symptomless depigmented macules of varying shapes and sizes develop on previously pigmented skin. It is a cause of great concern because of the widespread fear of leprosy with which it is often confused.

Vitiligo may be localised to one region, widespread or almost generalised but the iris does not lose its pigment. The degree of loss of pigment may vary from minimal to total. Melanocytes may still be present in the affected parts but have become non-functional. Hair in the affected parts may also lose its pigment.

The exposed parts (face, hands and feet) are more commonly affected. Vitiligo is seen in both sexes and in all ages.

Many cases of vitiligo are idiopathic and there may also be a family history of the condition. Auto-immune mechanisms and neurochemical factors are among the current hypotheses as to causation.

Some cases may be associated with trauma (for example, a grazing injury or bruise), ulcers, burns, sunburn, alopecia areata, infections (for example, leprosy), infestations with animal parasites (for example, onchodermatitis), metabolic or endocrine disorders (for example, diabetes mellitus, hyperthyroidism, hyperparathyroidism) and blood disorders (for example, Addison's pernicious anaemia).

Treatment

This is difficult and discouraging. Spontaneous repigmentation (complete or incomplete) may take place in some cases and make treatment unnecessary.

Drugs which have been found useful include:

(1) Meladinine tablets and paint (extract of an Egyptian lily: *Ammi majus*). This treatment held sway in the 1950s and 1960s but

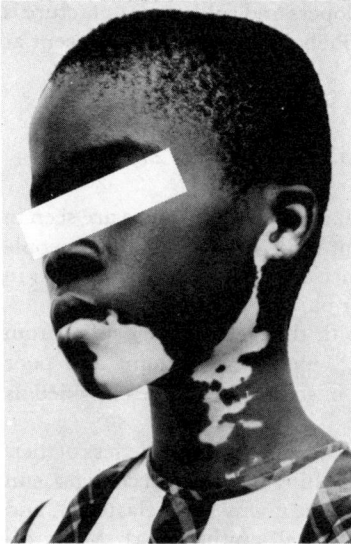

Figure 13.1   *(Left)* Vitiligo affecting the chin, neck and ear.
Figure 13.2   *(Right)* Vitiligo widespread on face, trunk and limbs.

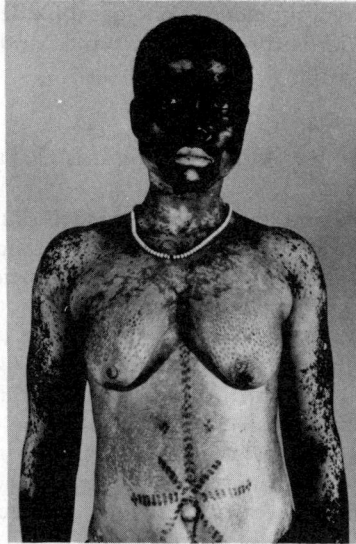

depigmentation after initial success was common.

(2) 8-Methoxypsoralen (methoxsalen) or trioxsalen (Trisoralen) tablets and paint. These have also been found effective in the treatment of vitiligo. The oral dose is 40–50 mg taken two hours before exposure to sunlight or ultraviolet light. Both drugs are expensive and difficult to obtain. Following administration, the skin should be exposed to graded sunlight or ultraviolet light.

(3) Fluorinated corticosteroid creams have been helpful in some cases.

Localised vitiligo can be covered cosmetically with 'covermark' or other tinted powders or creams to match the patient's skin.

The treatment of the underlying conditions in vitiligo associated with these conditions should be combined with local treatment of the vitiligo.

Differential diagnosis

Tuberculoid leprosy is associated with anaesthesia, and peripheral nerve thickening. Acquired leucoderma from monobenzyl ether of hydroquinone in photographic developers and rubber manufacture is localised to the fingers and hands. Piebaldism is usually present at birth.

13.2   **Albinism** (figures 13.3 and 13.4 and plate 27)

Albinos lack melanin in their skin, hair and eyes. Albinos are seen in every racial stock, but they stand out most strikingly among people with dark pigmentation. The incidence of albinism appears higher in Southern Nigeria than in many other parts of Africa.

The first problem of albinos is with their eyes. They suffer from photophobia (shrinking from light), nystagmus, squint and poor vision which may be severe enough in some cases to be classified as blindness.

The major problem of albinos in the tropics is the proneness of their skin to damage by sunlight and the resulting train of skin changes: sun burn, freckles, lentigines, solar keratoses, tawny skin (elastosis), and skin cancer (squamous-cell and basal-cell epithelioma). Many albinos in the tropics develop skin cancer as early as in their teens, and die from it in their twenties or thirties unless adequate treatment is given. The life span of albinos is therefore shortened by this early development of skin cancer, mainly squamous-cell epithelioma. Some

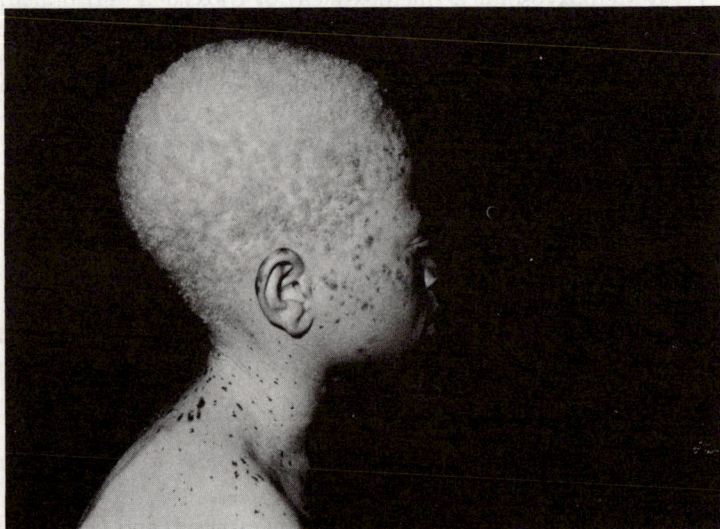

Figure 13.3   Albino child with lentigines on the face and neck.

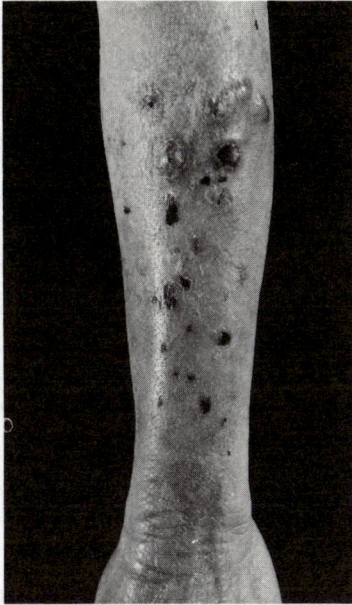

Figure 13.4 Albino showing lentigines, actinic keratoses and early
squamous-cell epithelioma on the forearm.

albinos also develop sarcoma (malignant connective-tissue tumour).

Albinos also suffer from the reaction of society to their condition.
Many of the native names for albinos are derisive. In spite of being of
normal intelligence, albinos endure much social snobbery which
along with poor vision, is responsible for their relatively poor achieve-
ment in life.

Inheritance of albinism

Oculocutaneous albinism is inherited as an autosomal recessive
genetic trait. Both parents of an albino must carry the genetic trait
even though they may be normally pigmented, just as both parents of
a sickler must carry the sickling trait even though they may not be
sicklers.

Various forms of albinism have been delineated: tyrosinase-
positive albinism, tyrosinase-negative albinism, yellow-mutant albinism, Hermansky–Pudlak syndrome, Cross syndrome and brown
albinism. Each involves a block in some locus in the synthesis of
melanin.

Care of albinos

Albinos should be registered as soon after birth as possible. As the albino child begins to go out in the sun every effort should be made to protect the skin against the sun, using protective skin lotions and creams and protective clothing including hats or other head-gear.

As the albino child begins to go to school, his eyes should be examined and any errors that can be corrected should be corrected to help him with his reading. Every encouragement should be given to help the child in school and he should be guided into productive occupations which will involve minimal exposure to sunlight.

In teenage and later, early skin changes should be treated early to guard against their developing into skin cancer. 5-Fluorouracil may be injected into the lesions or applied with or without occlusive dressing. If skin cancer develops, it should be treated promptly by surgery or with anti-cancer drugs.

13.3   Hyperpigmentation

Increase in skin pigmentation may be generalised due to the action of melanocyte-stimulating hormone (MSH) of the intermediate lobe of the pituitary gland. It may be seen in Addison's disease, Cushing's syndrome, Hodgkin's lymphomas, acromegaly, haemochromatosis, cirrhosis of the liver and administration of high doses of cortico-trophin (ACTH) which contains traces of MSH.

Localised hyperpigmentation may complicate acne vulgaris, on-chodermatitis, lichen planus, lichenified eczema, lichenified drug eruption, fixed drug eruption, contact dermatitis, pregnancy, proges-togens, photosensitivity, radiation treatment, neurofibromatosis, acanthosis nigricans, and the application of cosmetics.

Management of hyperpigmentation

In generalised hyperpigmentation, the underlying systemic disorder should be treated.

In localised hyperpigmentation, treatment is seldom necessary as the hyperpigmentation tends to fade after a variable period. Lotions or creams used to treat the underlying inflammation are usually sufficient.

Bleaching creams are not recommended as they tend to produce patch hypopigmentation. Some women will, however, be difficult to convince not to try bleaching creams on their own.

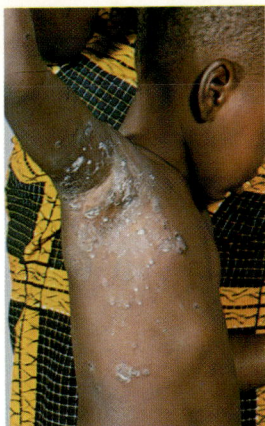

Plate 1

Impetigo contagiosum: broken vesicles and bullae, scabs and scales.

Plate 2

Bullous impetigo contagiosum.

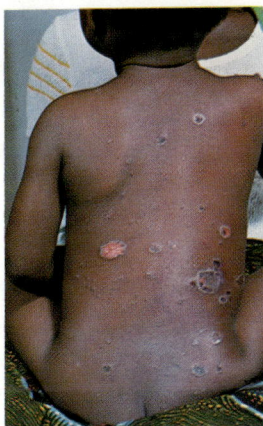

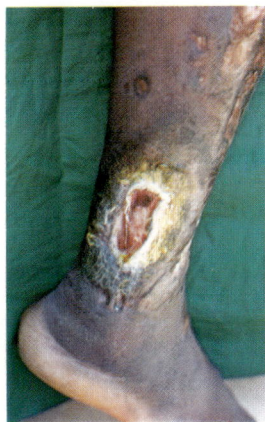

Plate 3

Chronic leg ulcer.

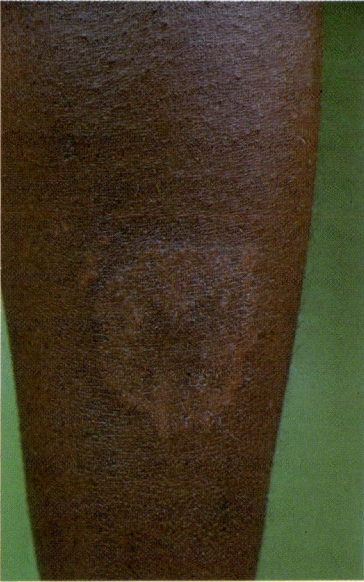

Plate 4
Tuberculoid leprosy.

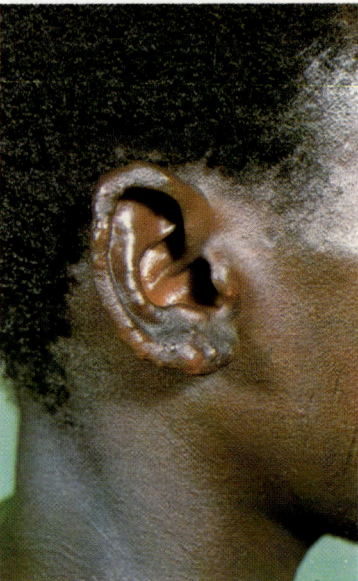

Plate 5
Lepromatous leprosy:
nodules on ear lobe.

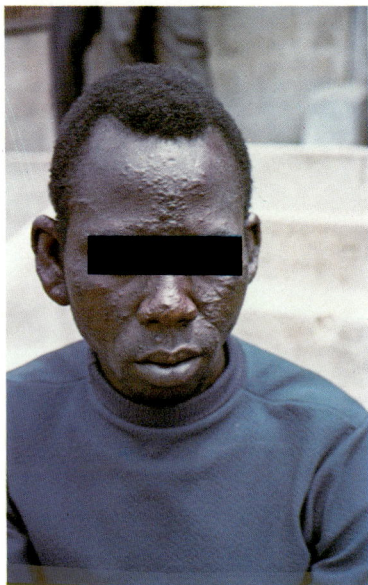

Plate 6

Lepromatous leprosy:
nodules on face and ear.

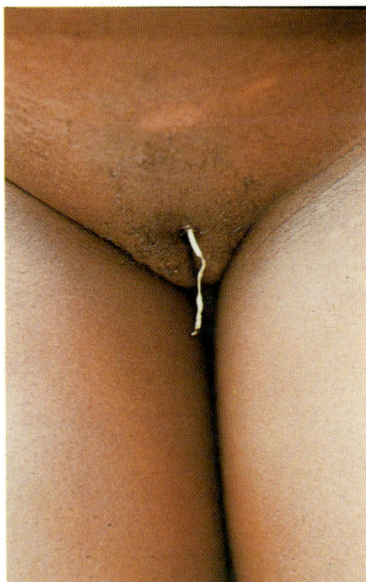

Plate 7

Guinea worm: unusual site.
Foot, ankle and lower leg
more common sites.

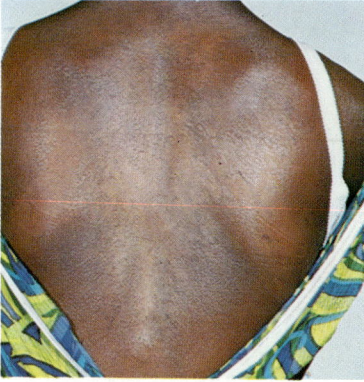

Plate 8

Tinea versicolor: sheets of brown scales in interscapular region.

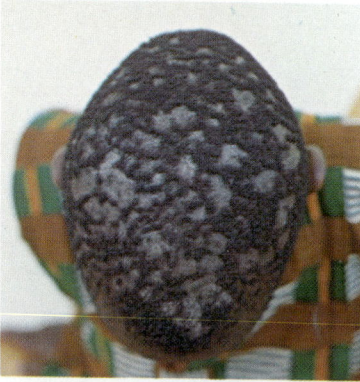

Plate 9

Tinea capitis: moth-eaten dry scaly lesions.

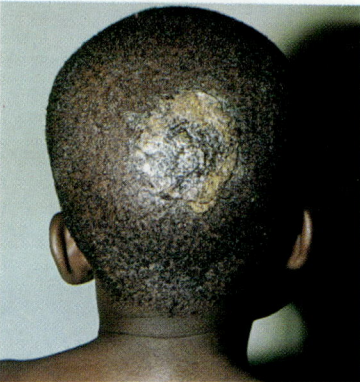

Plate 10

Kerion: scalp ringworm with inflammatory reaction and bacterial infection producing a boggy swelling.

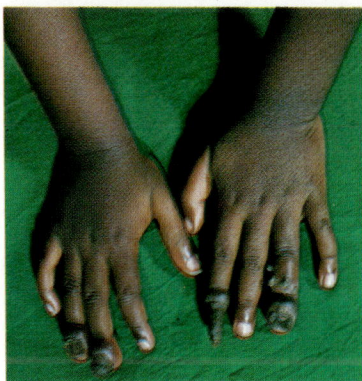

Plate 11

Tinea corporis: circinate
lesions.

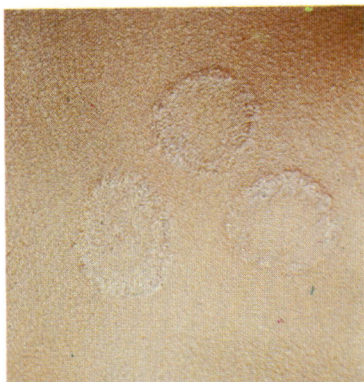

Plate 12

Cutaneous candidiasis:
granulomatous lesions from
chronic paronychia.

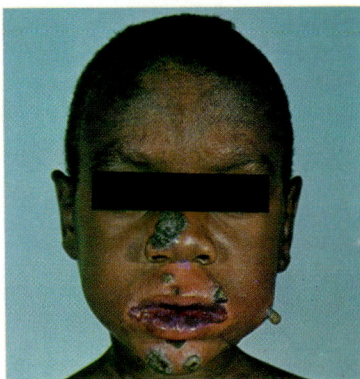

Plate 13

Cutaneous candidiasis:
erosion of lips and
granulomatous lesions on
face.

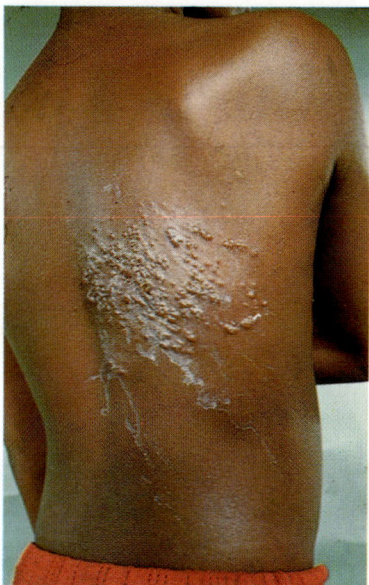

Plate 14

Herpes zoster: clusters of vesicles on the flank.

Plate 15

Herpes zoster: clusters of vesicles over the cutaneous distribution of mandibular division of the trigeminal nerve.

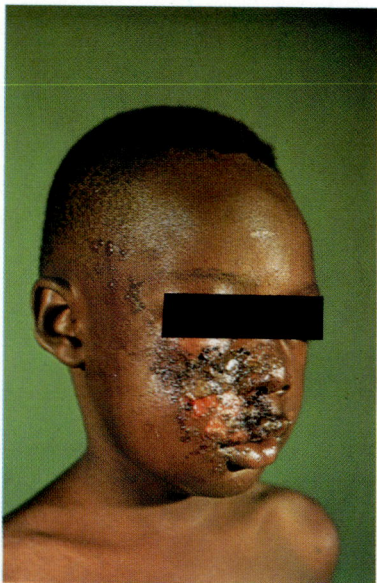

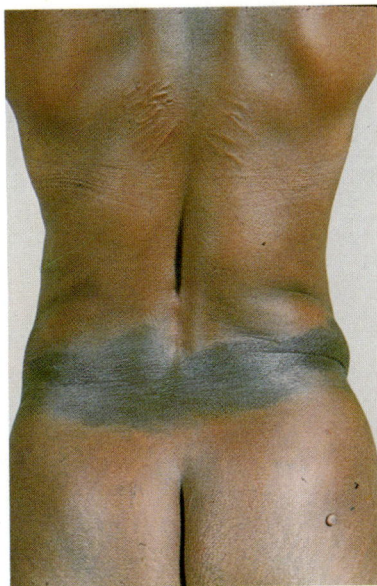

Plate 16

Allergic contact dermatitis due to rubber band.

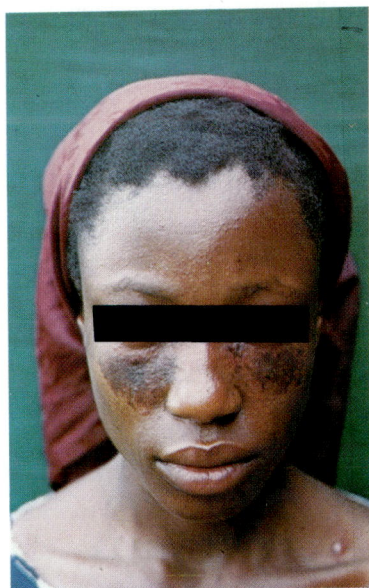

Plate 17

Dermatitis medicamentosa.

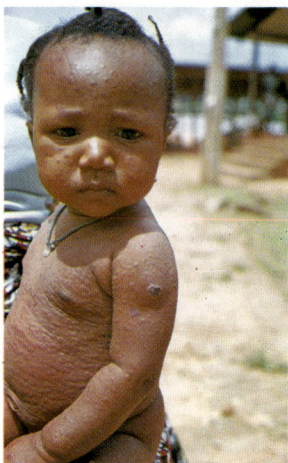

Plate 18

Eczema vaccinatum: exacerbation of atopic eczema following smallpox vaccination.

Plate 19

Flexural eczema.

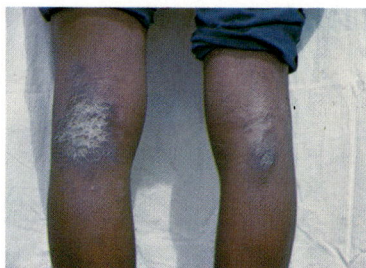

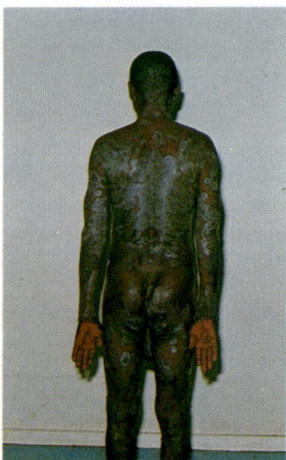

Plate 20

Lichen planus: widespread slaty-grey papules and plaques.

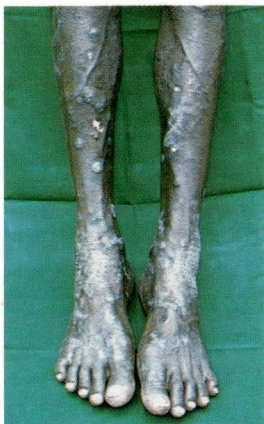

Plate 21

Lichen planus: hypertrophic
verrucose plaques.

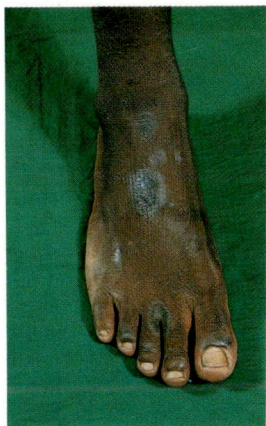

Plate 22

Erythema multiforme: discoid
pigmented lesions.

Plate 23

Fixed drug eruption: circinate
bluish-black macules on the thigh.

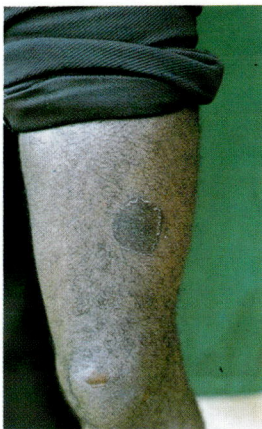

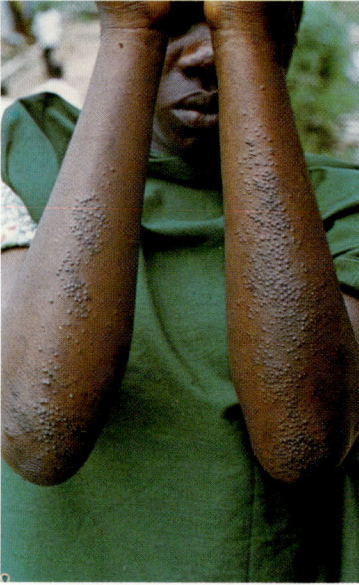

Plate 24

Phrynoderma: spinous papular eruption on elbows and forearms.

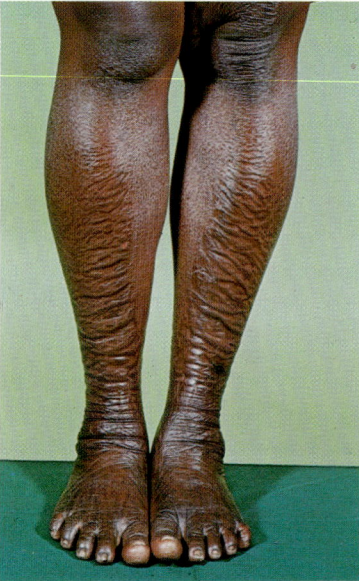

Plate 25

Pellagra: flaky eruption on lower legs.

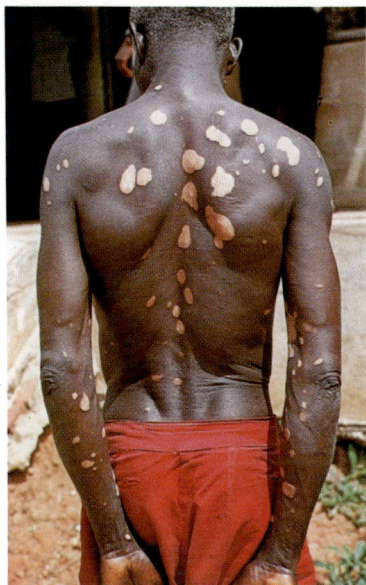

Plate 26

Vitiligo: multiple depigmented macules on the trunk and arms.

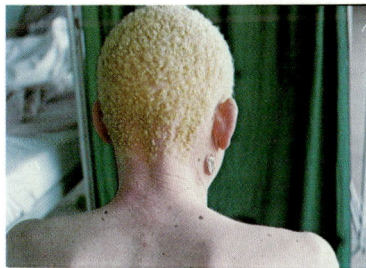

Plate 27

Albino with early skin cancer on the cheek.

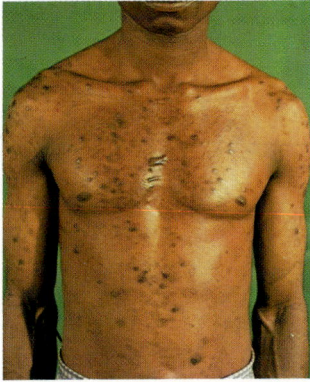

Plate 28

Acne vulgaris: papules, pustules, cysts, scars and keloids.

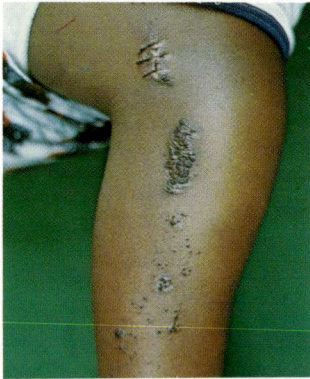

Plate 29

Keratotic naevus: warty epidermal tumour, linear in pattern.

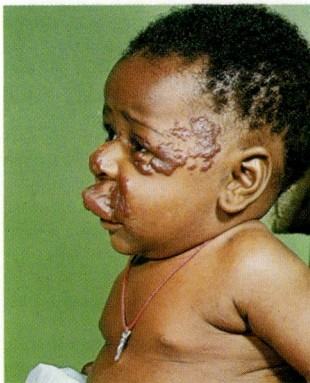

Plate 30

Cavernous haemangioma: purplish soft lesions on face and lips.

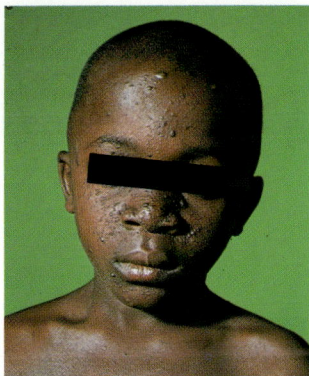

Plate 31

Cavernous haemangioma: dusky spongy lesions on leg, infected and ulcerated.

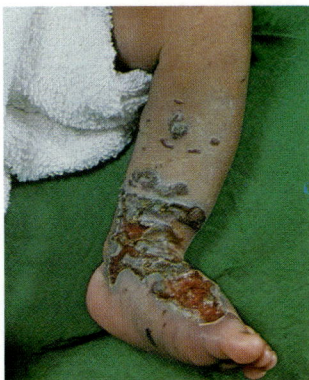

Plate 32

Adenoma sebaceum: papular tumours on the face. Father similarly affected.

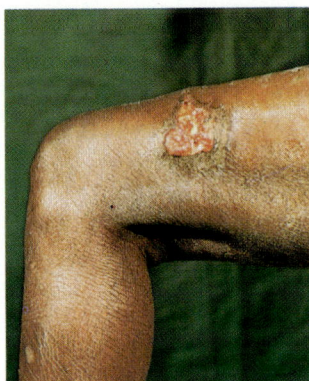

Plate 33

Squamous cell epithelioma in a normally pigmented person.

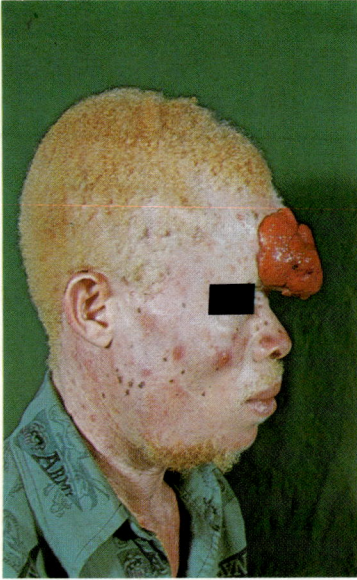

Plate 34

Horn-like fungating squamous cell epithelioma in an albino.

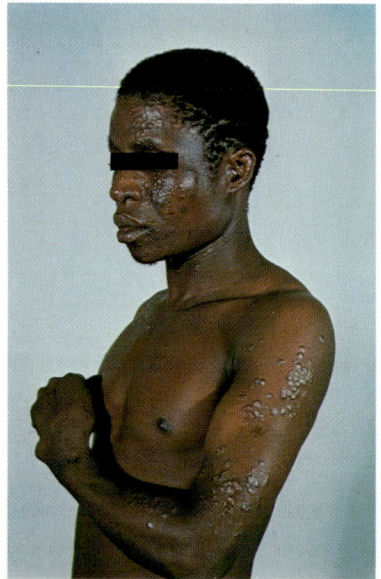

Plate 35

Lupus vulgaris: granulomatous and scarring lesions on the face and arms.

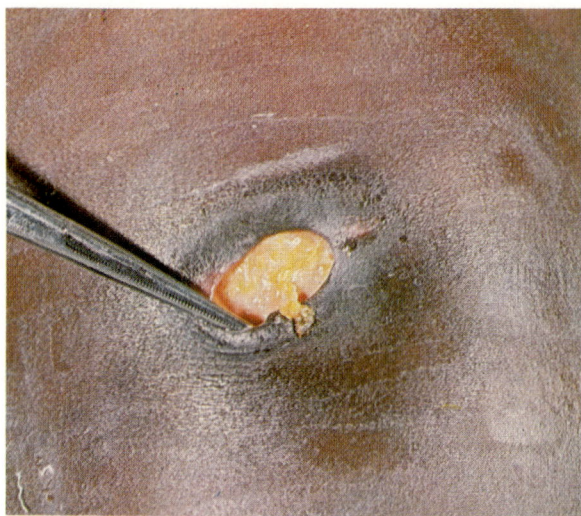

Plate 36

Buruli ulcer: chronic ulcer with undermined edges,
caused by *Mycobacterium ulcerans*.

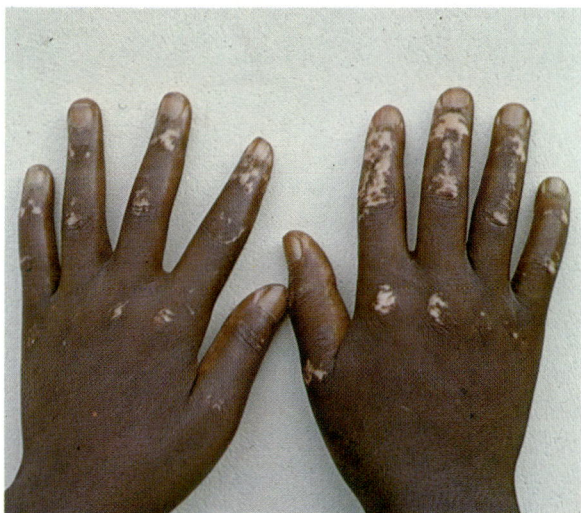

Plate 37

Scleroderma: skin bound down to hands and fingers.
Associated vitiligo.

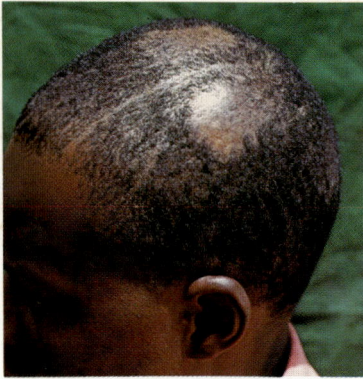

Plate 38

Trichotillomania: compulsive hair pulling due to psychological stress.

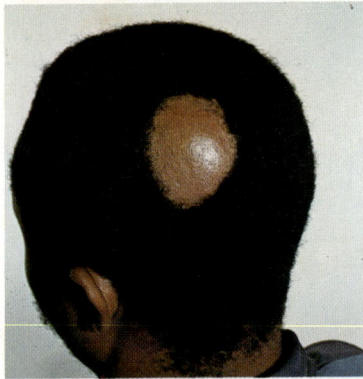

Plate 39

Alopecia areata.

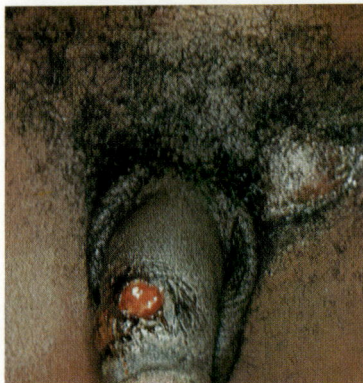

Plate 40

Granuloma inguinale.

14 Acne Vulgaris

Acne vulgaris (pimples) is so common among adolescents and young adults as to be considered almost physiological. A number of factors that are on the upswing in this age range increase the chances of acne developing. Androgens produced by both males and females stimulate sebaceous gland enlargement, increased sebum production and increased keratinisation near the mouths of the hair follicles. Progesterone also stimulates sebaceous gland activity. Propionibacterium acnes, resident in the hair follicles helps to produce fatty acids from sebum.

Friction, inflammation, secondary bacterial infection and tension all help to aggravate acne vulgaris.

Management of acne vulgaris is directed towards reversing or minimising the effects of these known triggers or aggravating factors.

Acne vulgaris is the ordinary pimple which is seen commonly in teenagers and young adults. In this age it is almost physiological, but clinical acne vulgaris is an inflammatory disorder involving the pilo-sebaceous follicles and surrounding tissues.

14.1 How common is acne vulgaris?

Acne is very common in teenage and if every teenage face is scrutinised for the mildest degree of acne, an incidence close to 100 per cent can be obtained. But only a small proportion of people with pimples have a problem sufficient to bring them to the doctor.

Acne starts in early adolescence with a peak incidence in girls at 14–15 years and in boys at 16–17 years. It may occur in both sexes well into the twenties. Pimples may get better or worse or may remain unchanged during pregnancy. The tendency to develop acne is inherited, and the condition is commoner in some families than in others.

14.2 Distribution (figures 14.1 and 14.2 and plate 28)

An oily or greasy skin is one of the early signs of acne vulgaris. Acne vulgaris of varying grades (subclinical, mild, moderate or severe) is seen on the face, front of chest, shoulders and upper back. The

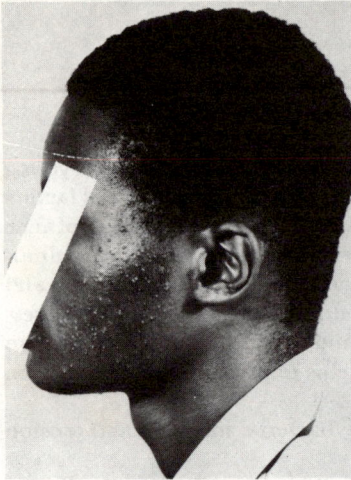

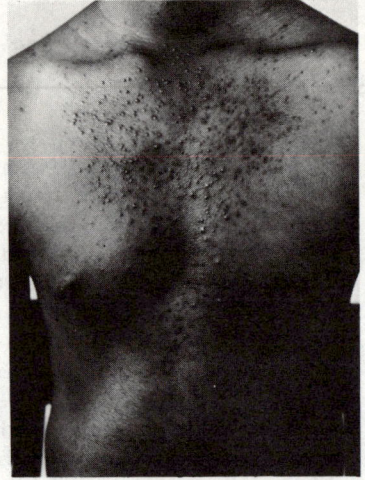

Figure 14.1   *(Left)* Acne vulgaris: papules and pustules on the face.

Figure 14.2   *(Right)* Acne vulgaris: papules and pustules on the chest.

common lesions seen on these sites include small papules which the patient may not have noticed, obvious papules consisting of comedones ('yellow heads' or 'black heads'), large papules or pustules, and complicated lesions such as nodules, cellulitis, abscesses, cysts, scars, or keloids.

14.3   How acne vulgaris is produced

Acne vulgaris usually begins around adolescence when sex hormones, mainly androgens but also progesterone stimulate sebaceous glands to enlarge and produce more sebum. Sebum is a mixture of fats, fatty acids, wax alcohols, glycerol and sterols. Bacteria which live in hair follicles especially *Propionibacterium acnes* produces a lipase which splits the main contents of sebum to produce fatty acids. Fatty acids irritate the follicular wall, and keratinisation at the mouths of the hair follicles is increased. The sebum accumulates behind the blocked follicles, solidifies, and becomes the oily 'yellow head' or 'black head'.

The build-up of more sebum behind the 'black heads' pushes them to the surface as pimples.

Complications may follow damage to the follicular wall, irritation and inflammation of surrounding tissue, and bacterial infection. All these can be made worse by frequent pressing or picking of the pimples.

14.4 Factors which may make acne worse

In spite of the popular belief that chocolates, sweets, nuts, fats and carbohydrates can make acne worse, there is no scientific proof that these specific items of food by themselves worsen acne.

Trauma and friction

Frequent pressing or picking, rubbing, scrubbing with medicated soaps, or pressure from tight clothing can damage the distended hair follicles and increase the inflammation. Worse than this, infection can spread to the cavernous sinus and cause a severe or fatal thrombosis.

Cosmetics

Cosmetics such as cleansing creams contain chemicals which may damage the hair follicles and aggravate acne.

Hormones and emotion

In some teenage girls or young women, acne may flare up in mid-cycle or premenstrually. In others acne may get worse during pregnancy. Adrenal and ovarian androgens are probably responsible for these exacerbations which may also reflect emotional changes. Treatment with systemic corticosteroids may light up smouldering acne.

14.5 Treatment and management

Reassurance

The natural history of most mild cases is that they clear up on their own by late teenage or a little later. For patients with this type, what is needed is confident reassurance and advice to avoid known factors (friction and cosmetics) which can make acne worse. Any foods which the patient has noticed as having worsened the acne should be avoided.

Objectives of specific treatment

Because there is no specific aetiology, specific treatment is aimed at controlling the three main factors in production of acne:

 (1) Sebum production and accumulation.
 (2) Bacterial population of the hair follicles. *Propionibacterium acnes, Pityrosporum ovale* and coagulase negative cocci.
 (3) Keratinisation of the follicular epithelium.

Control of sebum production or accumulation

Systemic administration of antiandrogens, usually oestrogens can reduce sebum production. The one in common use where appropriate is the oral contraceptive containing oestrogen and progesterone. It cannot be used in males because of its feminising effect. In females with severe acne, it may be used but its adverse side effects must be weighed against its benefit in acne. It may upset the rhythm of menstruation, cause vascular disorders, or predispose to cancer.

Benzol peroxide 5–10 per cent in a gel base applied locally breaks down the comedones (yellow heads and black heads) and also has antibacterial properties. Frequent washing with soap and water can help degrease the skin and lessen the accumulation of sebum.

Control of bacterial load

In acne vulgaris with pustules, the bacterial load can be controlled by prolonged administration of tetracycline or its derivatives 0.5–1 g daily, reduced after 4 weeks to 0.25–0.5 g daily. Erythromycin is also useful in similar doses.

Control of excessive keratinisation of the hair follicles

Vitamin A in the form of tretinoin (Retin-A) lotion 0.05 per cent, or cream 0.05–0.1 per cent reduces keratinisation. It has irritant, drying and peeling properties. Combination of Retin-A cream and benzoyl peroxide gel, by applying them alternately during the day may improve the results. Salicylic acid is the third of the useful exfoliants.

Incision and drainage of pustules

Large boils should be incised and drained. Appropriate antibiotics should be given.

14.6   Oil acne

Petroleum oils, other mineral oils and some vegetable oils may provoke acneiform lesions on the limbs, trunk or face after prolonged contact with the skin.

14.7 **Rosacea**

This is a facial disorder characterised by recurrent flushing (erythema) of the face which ultimately results in persistent erythema and telangiectasia. Inflammatory papules and pustules develop later and may be mistaken for acne vulgaris papules and pustules hence the old name of 'acne rosacea'. Rosacea develops later in life than acne vulgaris.

The persistent erythema, and papules and pustules of rosacea are more central on the face than those of acne vulgaris. Hot beverages and alcohol are thought to worsen rosacea lesions. Ocular lesions may also develop in chronic rosacea, presenting as blepharitis, keratoconjunctivitis or iritis.

A rare and disfiguring complication of rosacea is rhinophyma, a bullous deformity of the nose from gross sebaceous gland hyperplasia.

Treatment

Chlortetracycline or tetracycline 250 mg daily for about three months produces good results. Ichthammol 2 per cent in zinc cream or sulphur 2 per cent in cream base are among the useful older remedies. Hydrocortisone cream and benzoyl peroxide gel are also helpful but the condition seldom clears up completely. Beverages and drinks which produce flushing of the face should be avoided.

15 Tumours of the Skin

Among the many benefits bestowed on man by the large size, wide coverage and easy accessibility of the skin is that of its ready availability for the development of the science of oncology in a tumour-conscious and cancer-fearing world. The onset and progress of skin tumours can be observed more readily than those of any other organ. Tumours can be produced experimentally using known or suspected carcinogens. Ablation of some skin tumours can be achieved completely by excision, chemotherapy, cryotherapy or irradiation.

Tumours of the skin are virtually innumerable. They range from harmless virus-induced warts and molluscum contagiosum to invasive squamous-cell carcinoma and lethal nodular malignant melanoma.

An attempt at exhaustive classification or enumeration can be counter-productive. What is important is a simple guide to distinguishing harmless, benign, potentially dangerous and frankly life-threatening tumours, one from another. It is also important to be able to reassure confidently, give cosmetic treatment, offer current and effective therapy or refer difficult or dangerous tumours to centres with the expertise to handle them.

For such a large and vast organ as the skin which is made up of a wide variety of tissues, and which is influenced by genetic factors and exposed to numerous tumour-inducing stimuli in nature, the chances of development of tumours are well-nigh limitless.

Tumours of the skin include neoplasms, hyperplasias, over-growths and malformations of epithelial, melanocytic, mesodermal, and lymphoreticular cells. Tumours in the skin may also arise from leukaemia or the lymphomas, or as secondaries from neoplasms of the viscera.

Tumours may be completely benign, potentially malignant, pre-malignant or malignant. In a cancer-conscious world, therefore, it is important to be able to distinguish clinically or histologically between the tumours which are dangerous to life and those which are not.

A malignant melanoma which grows wildly, metastasises widely and kills the patient is obviously malignant. So is an invasive squamous-cell epithelioma in an albino.

A Paget's disease of the nipple with a crusting and scaling, retraction of the nipple and a serous or blood-stained discharge is pre-malignant. So is an actinic keratosis with a dusky scaly plaque and a horny top.

A pigmented (melanocytic) naevus on the hand or foot or external genitalia which itches and darkens is potentially malignant. So is a very chronic leg ulcer.

Skin tags, capillary haemangioma, seborrhoeic keratosis, and multiple neurofibromatosis are all benign.

The distinctions between the various tumours in terms of danger to life are not always clear-cut. Clinical evidence of distant metastases, haematogenous or lymphatic spread, local invasiveness, and histological evidence of increased mitosis, incomplete differentiation, abnormal differentiation, abnormal maturation and abnormal cellular function and organisation all have to be considered in determining the benignity or malignancy of each tumour.

15.1 Benign tumours

Skin tags (figure 15.1)

These are small soft sessile or pedunculated skin-coloured or hyperpigmented outgrowths of the skin found on the neck, trunk or limbs in

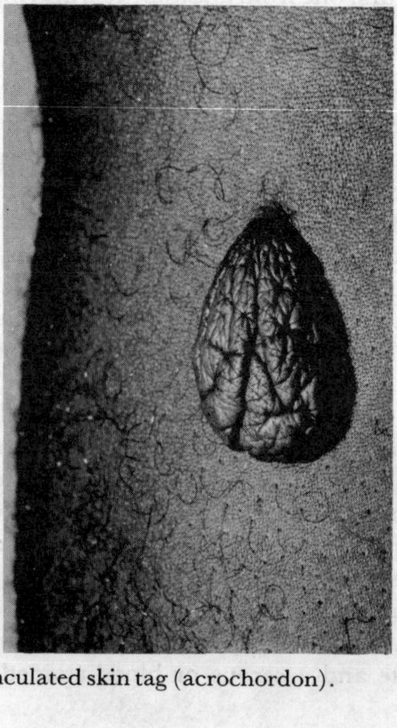

Figure 15.1 Pedunculated skin tag (acrochordon).

middle-aged or elderly people. In some women skin tags may prolifer-
ate during pregnancy or menopause.

Treatment Skin tags may be tied off with ligature and left to drop off
after some days. They may also be removed by curetting or diathermy
under local anaesthesia.

Blue naevus

This is a bluish or bluish-black macule or plaque which is present at
birth or appears later. The common sites are lumbar region and
buttocks, but other parts of the trunk or limbs may be involved.

Blue naevus is a developmental defect in which some melanocytes
are arrested in the dermis during their migration from the neural crest
to their normal destination in the basal layer of the epidermis. It is
sometimes called Mongolian blue spot.

Treatment This is seldom necessary. If the naevus is raised or nodular,
it may be excised.

Melanocytic naevus ('mole')

A naevus is a developmental defect of the skin the abnormality being
derived from melanocytic or vascular or other tissue.

A melanocytic naevus is a pigmented tumour formed by melanocytes proliferating at the dermo-epidermal junction and migrating to
the dermis. Melanocytic naevi look bluish or bluish black. They may
be present at birth, or may continue to appear during childhood and
early adult life. They tend to be less in old age. Melanocytic naevi may
present in the following forms:

(1) Congenital pigmented naevus. This is usually present at birth,
    is extensive with irregular surface, may be hairy, and has a
    tendency to malignant change to malignant melanoma.
(2) Compound naevus. This is large and dark with an irregular
    surface. It may become mammilated or papillomatous.
(3) Neuroid naevus. This type incorporates Schwann cells in the
    dermis and may be domed or pedunculated.
(4) Pigmented hairy epidermal naevus (Becker's naevus). This is a
    dark irregular and hairy naevus developing on the upper trunk
    and shoulders in adolescence or early adult life.
(5) Naevus of Ota. This is an oculo-cutaneous naevus affecting the
    face and iris.

Complications of naevi Inflammation, haemorrhage or thrombosis may occur in various types of melanocytic naevi, but transformation to malignant melanoma is the most serious complication. This malignant transformation is usually heralded by irritation, increase in pigmentation, bleeding or ulceration in an existing melanocytic naevus.

Capillary haemangioma *(port-wine naevus)*

This is a flat purplish or dusky stain which may be visible at birth or may appear in the first month or later. It is a developmental abnormality of small dermal blood vessels and may range from a few millimetres to several centimetres in diameter. It may be circular, ovoid or irregular in shape. It may increase in size as the child grows and may or may not fade in later life.

The common sites are the face, neck and upper trunk, but other sites and the muco-cutaneous junctions may be involved. The lesions may be few or numerous.

Treatment This is disappointing. Cover marks matched to the complexion of the individual may be used to conceal the blemish.

Cavernous haemangioma *(strawberry naevus)* (figure 15.2 and plates 30 and 31)

This is a fleshy purple or dusky tumour which may be visible in the first few days or weeks of birth as a tiny reddish spot resembling an insect bite. It is a developmental abnormality of dermal blood vessels.

It appears commonly on the face but may be seen on any part of the body. A haemangioma on the face or neck tends to increase in size as the child cries or strains. The tumour is soft and compressible. When it is small it blanches on pressure.

Complications include infection, thrombosis, haemorrhage, ulceration and scarring. Some of the tumours may disappear spontaneously in the first few years.

Treatment Because some cavernous haemangiomata involve spontaneously it is reasonable to observe small uncomplicated tumours and reassure the parents of the child. Photographs every 3–6 months may be taken to record the progress. Large, or infected or complicated tumours may call for more active treatment.

Systemic corticosteroids have been found useful in quickening resolution. Carefully regulated superficial X-ray treatment may be

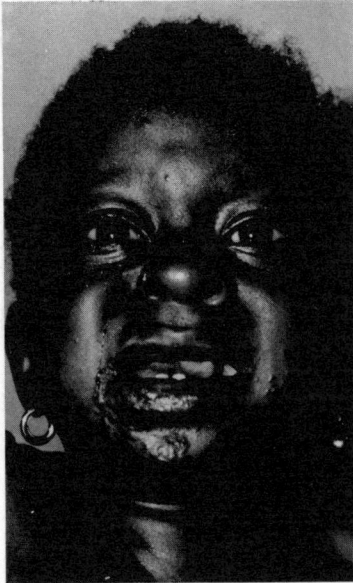

Figure 15.2 Cavernous haemangioma on face.

used. Carbon dioxide snow can be used to freeze some tumours. Plastic surgery may be called for usually after the age of five years when the maximum spontaneous resolution should have been achieved.

Lymphangiomata (figures 15.3 and 15.4)

These are boggy skin-coloured tumours or clusters of glistening papules or nodules or lymph filled vesicles usually in parts of the body where the skin is rather loose. They appear in childhood or later. The tumours may be infected and may discharge clear or offensive fluid.

Lymphangioma circumscriptum is the commonest type. It appears as a boggy tumour in the axilla, shoulder, waist, thigh or other parts. There may be associated haemangioma and the vesicles may discharge blood-stained fluid.

Treatment This is difficult and even a deep excision may be followed by a recurrence.

Seborrhoeic keratosis (*Seborrhoeic wart*)

This is a pigmented tumour of epidermal cells seen usually in the elderly. The tumours are usually numerous and appear in parts of the

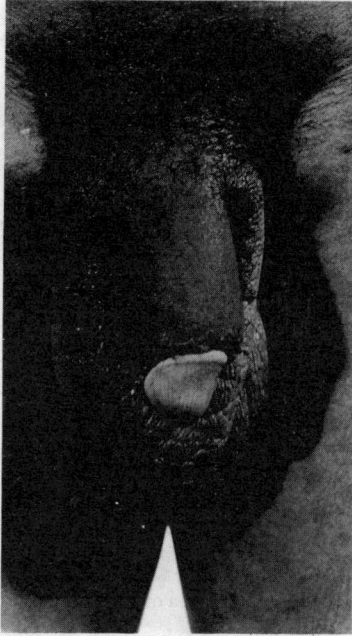

Figure 15.3   Lymphangioma of scrotum with oedema of penis.

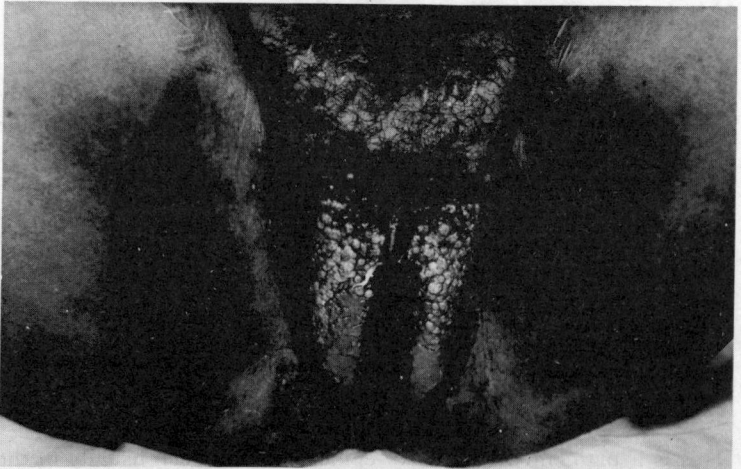

Figure 15.4   Lymphangioma of the vulva.

body rich in sebaceous glands – face, trunk, arms, hands. Some of the lesions may become pedunculated.

Treatment Seborrhoeic keratosis are easily removed by curetting, freezing, cautery or diathermy.

Granuloma telangiectaticum *(granuloma pyogenicum)* (figure 15.5)

This is a small rapidly growing reddish or dusky tumour at the site of a minor injury, for example, a cut during shaving, an accidental bite on the lip, a pin prick or a scratch.

It grows rapidly within a few days to a few weeks into a sessile or pedunculated nodule which bleeds readily on pressure or injury.

Treatment A sessile tumour may be ligated with a suture and left to drop off. Other tumours may be treated by diathermy or excision under local anaesthesia.

Adenoma sebaceum (plate 32)

This is a developmental dysplasia inherited as an autosomal domi-

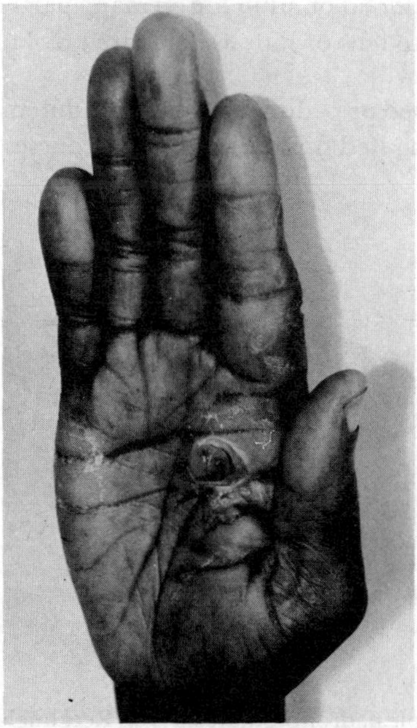

Figure 15.5 Granuloma telangiectaticum on the palm.

nant gene and affecting tissues of the skin, eyes, brain, kidneys, heart and lungs.

The skin lesions include brown or pink papules on the cheeks and nose, periungual fibromata and brown slightly raised macules on the trunk. These are seen in childhood or adult life.

Epilepsy and mental retardation are seen in the majority of patients with these skin lesions.

Treatment Little can be done about the visceral involvement but epilepsy should be treated with phenytoin sodium (Epanutin) or other standard drugs for the control of epilepsy. The tumours on the face can be removed by diathermy.

Multiple neurofibromatosis *(von Recklinghausen's disease of the skin)* (figure 15.6)

This is a neuro-cutaneous abnormality inherited as an autosomal dominant gene.

Skin lesions consist of:

(1) Soft fleshy skin-coloured or dark papules or nodules erupting during childhood or adult life on many parts of the body. These may run into tens or hundreds. Flare up of tumours may occur in pregnancy.
(2) Dome-shaped or pedunculated or pendulous large tumours.
(3) Diffuse elongated tumours along the courses of nerves.

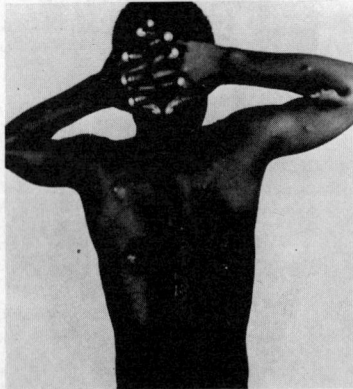

Figure 15.6   Multiple neurofibromatosis (von Recklinghausen's disease of the skin). Soft fleshy tumours on the trunk and limbs.

(4) Hyperpigmented macules or plaques spattered all over the body (café au lait spots).
(5) Muco-cutaneous and oral papillomata.
(6) Neurological lesions include optic nerve gliomas, intracranial tumours, spinal cord and peripheral nerve tumours.

Treatment Diathermy or excision of painful or disfiguring lesions. Control of epilepsy or neurosurgery if a tumour is the cause.

15.2   Pre-malignant tumours

These are tumours or skin conditions which if left untreated in time may become malignant.

Solar keratosis *(actinic keratosis)*

This presents as fixed erythema or telangiectasia followed by scaling, plaque formation or cutaneous horns. The common sites are the exposed parts – forehead, cheeks, temples, nose, ears, lips, sides of neck, dorsa of hands.

The high risk individuals are albinos and fair-skinned individuals living and working outdoors in sunny climates.

Treatment 5-Fluorouracil 5 per cent cream or 1 per cent lotion in propylene glycol applied topically with or without occlusive dressing. Intra-lesional injection of 5-fluorouracil often gives a better result than topical application. Sunscreen lotions or creams should be applied as protection thereafter.

Cutaneous horn

This is a hard brown or dark overgrowth of neglected epidermal plaque which is shaped like a thorn or horn. It may undergo malignant transformation to a squamous-cell epithelioma after frequent trauma and inflammation.

Kaposi's multiple idiopathic haemorrhagic sarcoma (figures 15.7 and 15.8)

This is a rare slowly growing granulomatous tumour of angiomatous and fibroblastic elements, affecting the skin and subcutaneous tissues of the feet and legs, hands and forearms. Reddish, dusky or bluish-black nodules develop, and oedema and induration spread along the affected limbs. There is a tendency for the lesions to bleed or ulcerate and to be secondarily infected. Other parts of the body may be involved, and rarely lesions may develop in the gastrointestinal tract, liver, heart and lung. The condition may last for many years without the patient coming to any harm, but massive haemorrhage in affected internal organs may lead to death.

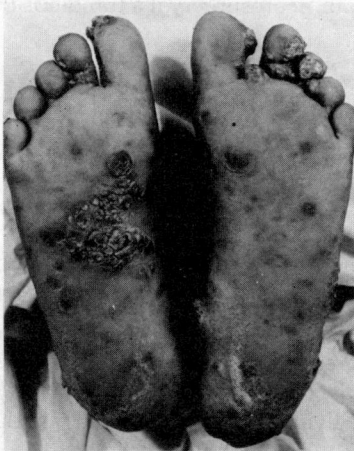

Figure 15.7   Kaposi's sarcoma: dusky keratotic nodules on the feet and toes.

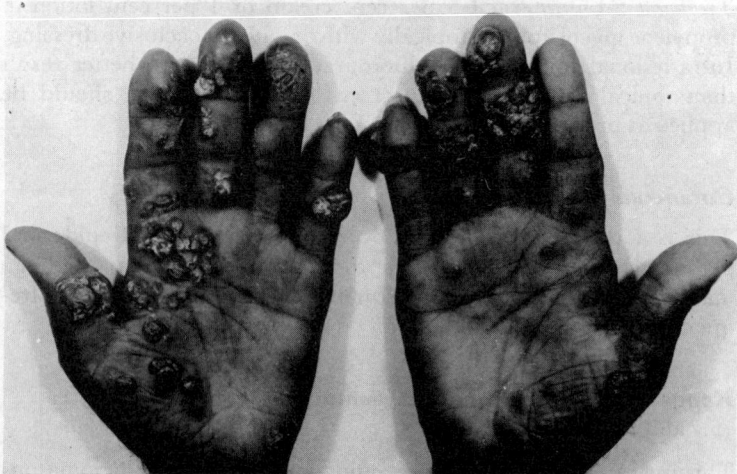

Figure 15.8   Kaposi's sarcoma: dusky keratotic nodules on the hands and fingers.

Histologically, proliferating capillary vessels and perivascular connective tissue cells predominate. There is proliferative endarteritis in the blood vessels, and inflammatory cells include macrophages, lymphocytes and spindle cells.

Differential diagnosis Elephantiasis, deep fungal infection, granuloma telangiectaticum and histiocytoma may be confused with Kaposi's sarcoma. Kaposi's sarcoma may co-exist with Hodgkin's lymphoma or with chronic lymphocytic leukaemia.

Treatment With small lesions, excision or radiotherapy may be sufficient, but recurrences are common.

Chemotherapy with cytotoxic drugs: methotrexate, cyclophosphamide (Endoxan), vinblastine sulphate or nitrogen mustard may bring about resolution of some lesions.

Paget's disease of the nipple

This is a chronic scaly and crusty erosion of the nipple and areola which may start with itching or burning and clear or serous or blood-stained discharge from the nipple. It is unilateral. The eczematous picture soon changes to give a marginated erosion with irregular raised edges and retraction of the nipple. A palpable induration may be felt in the underlying breast and carcinoma of the breast is a sequel.

Extramammary Paget's disease may be seen in other sites, for example, axilla, umbilicus, ano-genital region. In these areas, the tumour arises from apocrine glands.

Histologically, a carcinoma *in situ* is found, neoplastic cells spreading from the breast duct to involve the skin. Nucleated Paget cells with clear cytoplasm and no intercellular bridges lie among the prickle cells.

Differential diagnosis Eczema of the breast. This is usually bilateral, runs a shorter course and responds to treatment. Superficial basal-cell epithelioma.

Bowen's disease

This is a chronic scaly or crusted dusky plaque which may be seen on any part of the skin. After some years, the lesion becomes granular, raised and hyperkeratotic. It may then ulcerate. It has a tendency to be transformed to a squamous-cell carcinoma and to be associated with cancer of the gastrointestinals genito-urinary and respiratory systems.

Treatment In early stages, 5-fluorouracil applied topically over a period of weeks may produce regression of lesions. Later, curettage, electrodesiccation, superficial radiotherapy or excision may be required depending on the stage and extent of the lesions.

Mycosis fungoides

This is a chronic skin eruption, a three-stage cutaneous lymphoma, which starts with an ill-defined eczematous reaction, then develops infiltrated plaques and finally forms skin tumours and involves lymph nodes.

The disease usually starts in adult life as a non-specific eczematous eruption which fails to respond to the usual soothing creams and antihistamines. This is the premycotic stage. Later in the plaque stage, the eruption becomes dusky and itchy with infiltrated plaques. They may become exudative, infected or lichenified.

Many years later, in the tumour stage, tumescent nodules and larger soft tumours or fungating masses develop on the infiltrated plaques, and the lymph nodes become infiltrated.

Treatment of mycosis fungoides In early stages local application of fluorinated corticosteroids and systemic antihistamines offer relief but relapses follow.

5-Fluorouracil 5 per cent cream or Podophyllin resin 25 per cent may be applied locally.

Cytotoxic drugs: cyclophosphamide (Endoxan), vinblastine sulphate and methotrexate are useful in the tumour stage. Systemic corticosteroids may also be helpful.

Radiotherapy in fractionated doses may control some cases in the plaque and tumour stages. Freezing, cautery or diathermy may be preferable in some cases. Excision of circumscribed small tumours is usually successful.

15.3   Malignant tumours

These are the tumours with invasive properties and those to which the potentially malignant or pre-malignant tumours transform.

Basal-cell carcinoma *(rodent ulcer)*

This is a slowly growing carcinoma of the skin arising from the basal cells of the epidermis. It rarely metastasises, but is locally invasive and may erode muscle, cartilage and bone.

The typical tumour whose cells do not keratinise is a raised nodular plateau with a shiny surface and rolled edges. Basal-cell carcinoma may be single or multiple. Variations in form include the button-shaped type with an ulcerated centre, the crusted superficial type resembling an eczema, the nodular pigmented type resembling a melanoma, and the erosive type spreading over a wide area.

Basal-cell carcinoma is commonly seen on the head and neck particularly in the upper half and central parts of the face.

Sunlight is a major factor in causing the irritation and damage to basal cells of the epidermis. Basal-cell carcinoma are therefore commonest among fair-skinned people living in sunny climates especially if their work is outdoors.

Treatment If the tumour is properly localised, complete excision, with skin graft if necessary, will do.

In elderly people or for extensive tumours or those in sites where excision would be mutilating, radiotherapy is the best method provided the doses are well graduated and spread over some weeks.

For small superficial tumours, chemotherapy with 5-fluorouracil or methotrexate may be useful.

In expert hands, curettage of small or superficial lesions may be almost as effective as excision, with recurrence rate about the same with both methods.

Squamous-cell carcinoma (plates 33 and 34)

This is a rapidly growing tumour of the skin which may arise from normal, chronically irritated or damaged skin or mucosa. The tumour arises from the prickle cell layer of the epidermis or its appendages. Because of the ability of the prickle cells to keratinise, the early lesions of squamous-cell carcinoma are usually warty or hard.

The common sites are the face, scalp, ears, lips, mouth, external genitalia and limbs.

Sunlight is the commonest environmental carcinogen responsible for squamous-cell carcinoma which is the commonest skin tumour in albinos in the tropics. Other carcinogens include X rays, coal tar, mineral oils and arsenic.

Squamous-cell carcinoma may complicate chronic ulcers, lupus vulgaris, burn scars, lupus erythematosus, scleroderma.

Treatment For small or moderately large tumours, complete excision with or without skin graft is the treatment of choice. Radiotherapy using superficial X rays, radium or radioactive cobalt in special centres with radiotherapists and physicists can be useful.

Antimitotic drugs: 5-fluorouracil, cyclophosphamide and methotrexate given systemically can produce some resolution of some tumours.

Malignant melanoma (figure 15.9)

This is a rare very dangerous skin cancer which may arise from melanocytes, melanocytic naevi, apparently normal skin, mucosa, or the retina. Malignant melanoma grows rapidly, ulcerates, and metastasises through the lymphatics and blood stream to lymph nodes, liver, lungs, brain and nervous system, and bone marrow.

Malignant melanoma tends to grow laterally and slowly for some time before becoming more aggressive and growing rapidly downwards and metastasising.

Chemotherapy with cytotoxic drugs, arterial perfusion with cytotoxic drugs and immunotherapy have all been tried with variable success. Most tumours are pigmented but few are amelanotic.

Treatment Wide and deep excision with block dissection of the regional lymph nodes is necessary to limit its rapid progress. In advanced cases on the limbs, amputation may prove the only way of saving life.

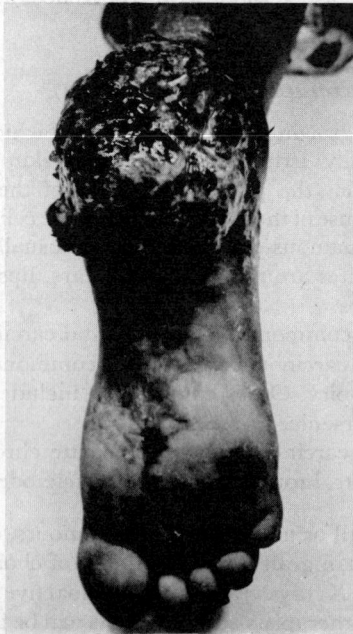

Figure 15.9 Malignant melanoma.

16 Miscellaneous Disorders

Some skin conditions which are afraid of being left out either because they have no dramatic photographs or because they are not in the 'top ten' as far as prevalence goes have found a home in this chapter. They are neither unimportant nor irrelevant and some illustrate landmarks in epidemiology, pathogenesis, clinical features, management or prognosis.

Two mycobacterial diseases, tuberculosis of the skin and Buruli ulcer show contrasting response to anti-tuberculous drugs.

Yaws though a vanishing disease illustrates the mimicry of treponemal diseases.

The connective tissue diseases show their localised features as well as their protean systemic manifestations.

The effects of physical pressure or emotional tension on the skin and its appendages are illustrated by keloids, keratoderma, hyperkeratosis and trichotillomania.

16.1 Tuberculosis of the skin

Considering the ravages of tuberculosis of the lungs, gut, kidneys, brain, spine, bones and other organs and tissues, cutaneous tuberculosis is comparatively rare in this environment. Cutaneous tuberculosis demonstrates varied immunological reactions of the skin to *Mycobacterium tuberculosis*.

Lupus vulgaris (plate 35) This is a chronic slowly ulcerative lesion which may cover wide areas of the face or other parts of the body, defying all common methods of ulcer treatment. The lesion is irregular with areas of healing and scarring and other areas of scaly or nodular plaques.

The tuberculin test is usually strongly positive, but tubercle bacilli are difficult to isolate from lesions.

Papulonecrotic tuberculide This is another form of cutaneous tuberculosis with widespread papular and pustular lesions on the face, trunk, and limbs. The lesions last for months or years, with a tendency to heal in parts and recur in others. The tuberculin test is strongly positive, but bacilli are seldom found in lesions.

Tuberculous adenitis Tuberculous adenitis with abscess or sinuses may develop in children especially in the neck or other folds. The tuberculin test is usually strongly positive. Bacilli may be found in biopsy material.

Papular tuberculide This may develop spontaneously or after BCG vaccination or tuberculin test. Lesions may be papular, necrotic or scarring. The tuberculin test is positive.

Verrucose tuberculosis usually presents as warty or verrucose papules or plaques following direct cutaneous inoculation in a strongly immune individual. The tuberculin test is strongly positive.

Scrofuloderma This is a form in which lymph node or bone lesions suppurate and sinus tracts lead to the skin surface. It is more common in children than in adults.

Erythema induratum (Bazin's disease) This presents as large dusky nodules on the calves, with a tendency to ulceration. The tuberculin test is strongly positive.

Treatment of cutaneous tuberculosis

The treatment of all forms of cutaneous tuberculosis should be the same as for systemic or visceral tuberculosis with a combination of two of the first line drugs. Streptomycin 0.5–1 g daily or 3 times weekly. Isoniazid 150–300 mg daily. Ethambutol 400 mg t.i.d. The duration of treatment should be 18–24 months. Rifampicin 300–600 mg daily in combination with isoniazid can shorten the period of treatment considerably.

16.2 *Mycobacterium ulcerans* infection *(Buruli ulcer)* (plate 36)

This is a chronic ulceration of the skin caused by an atypical acid fast bacillus called *Mycobacterium ulcerans.*

The condition has been described in various tropical and subtropical regions including Australia, Buruli in Uganda, Nigeria, Zaire, Malaysia, Indonesia, New Guinea, Peru and Mexico.

Clinical features

The condition usually starts as a dusky, firm, painless skin nodule or induration which breaks down after some weeks or months. A necrotic ulcer develops which extends deeply under the skin leaving very undermined overhanging edges. The ulcer is shallow with a granular floor but a probe can be pushed deeply on all sides. The exposed parts of the body are more commonly affected than the covered parts.

The ulcer may extend widely or be accompanied by satellite ulcers. Healing is very slow and secondary pyogenic infection may complicate the ulcers.

Diagnosis

This is based on the history, the pre-ulcerative lesions and ulcers. An atypical acid fast bacilli may be demonstrated from swabs or in biopsy specimens.

Treatment

Excision of ulcer with skin grafting is usually necessary. Antituberculous drugs are usually ineffective but rifampicin has shown some promise.

Trimethoprim + sulphamethoxazole (Septrin) has been found useful in some cases and has made mutilating surgery unnecessary. BCG vaccination in endemic areas has been found to offer reasonable protection.

16.3 Yaws

This is a contagious skin disease which presents as crusted, ulcerative or fungating papules or nodules. Unless it is promptly diagnosed and treated, it usually passes through primary, secondary and tertiary stages and may end up with deformation of the feet, legs, arms or face.

Causal organism

Yaws is caused by a spirochaete, *Treponema pertenue*, which resembles *Treponema pallidum*, the spirochaete which causes syphilis. Yaws is however not a sexually transmitted disease. It occurs mainly in childhood. Its late stages (secondary and tertiary) do not affect the cardiovascular or the central nervous system, and the disease is not transmitted to the unborn child.

Incidence

Yaws is a disease of underdevelopment, poverty and crowded rural living. It is found predominantly in the hot and humid equatorial belt, especially in parts of Central and West Africa. The extreme sensitivity of the causal organism to penicillin and the sustained WHO campaign with mass treatment with penicillin has eliminated yaws in all but a few inaccessible rural pockets.

Clinical features

The source of infection is usually the open yaws lesion which is teeming with spirochaetes. These reach the skin of an unaffected person through close personal contact and enter through broken skin: cut, scratch, bite or wound.

After an incubation period of a few weeks, an erythematous or dusky papule develops. This grows into an ulcerated nodule covered with scabs and crusts. This is the 'mother yaws' and may grow into a fungating mass and be surrounded by smaller papules and nodules. There may be associated regional lymphadenitis and fever, joint pains and malaise.

The 'mother yaws' usually heals spontaneously, leaving a scar. But about two or three months later, a widespread crop of papules erupts. These grow into ulcerated nodules covered with scabs and crusts. These are called the 'daughter yaws', and may be associated with constitutional disturbances and lymphadenopathy. They may last for months or years and then heal, leaving scars.

The tertiary stage of yaws is characterised by hyperkeratosis or keratoderma of palms and soles, nodular and ulcerative lesions on the skin, involvement of the bones of the legs or arms, or destruction of the nasal cartilage and other cartilaginous or bony tissues of the face.

Diagnosis

This is based on the finding of characteristic primary, secondary or tertiary lesions, in an endemic area. Laboratory findings include:

(1) *Treponema pertenue* in smears from primary or secondary lesions, identified by dark-ground examination.
(2) Serological tests: Kahn test; treponemal immobilisation test; complement fixation tests.
(3) Histopathology – epidermal changes, including acanthosis, papillomatosis and microabscesses are more striking than dermal changes which consist mainly of cellular infiltrates but without the endothelial proliferation seen in syphilis.

Differential diagnosis

Conditions which may be confused with yaws include:

(1) Secondary syphilis. Mucosal lesions, other stigmata of secondary syphilis, and the positive VDRL test should confirm this.
(2) Pinta – this shows more severe pigmentary changes on shins, arms and other parts.
(3) Leishmaniasis–Leishman–Donovan bodies can be isolated.
(4) Plantar warts.
(5) Plantar hyperkeratosis.

Treatment

Penicillin is very effective. A single dose of benzathine penicillin or PAM (penicillin G in oil with 2 per cent aluminium monostearate) 1.2–2.4 megaunits according to age or procaine penicillin 400,000–800,000 units on alternate days for 4 doses.

Prophylactic measures

Improving living conditions, minimising contact with infected persons, prompt treatment of diagnosed cases, and mass treatment with penicillin of people in endemic areas have reduced the incidence markedly. These measures consistently applied should eliminate the disease.

16.4 Pinta

This is another spirochaetal disease. It is caused by *Treponema carateum* which resembles the causal organisms of syphilis and yaws.

Pinta has a restricted geographical distribution: Central and South America.

Clinical features

Like syphilis and yaws, pinta evolves in three stages. Like yaws it affects the skin and occasionally the lymph nodes, but does not involve the cardiovascular or nervous system. Infection is usually by close personal contact especially in childhood.

In the primary stage, dusky or erythematous macules or plaques develop on the face, arms, legs or other exposed parts. In the secondary phase, months or years later, widespread mottled hypopigmentation or scaling develops in the exposed parts.

In the tertiary stage which may merge with the secondary stage, variable depigmentation and hyperpigmentation affects the exposed parts and bony prominences in covered parts. Scaling, thickening of the skin or atrophy of the skin on the shins and over bony prominences may result. Lymphadenitis may also develop.

Diagnosis

This is based on the clinical picture of the various stages. *Treponema carateum* may be isolated in smears from primary or secondary lesions examined under dark ground examination as in yaws. Serological tests which may be positive include Kahn test, Wasserman test, and VDRL test.

Differential diagnosis

Conditions which may mimic the pigmentary changes of pinta include yaws, onchodermatitis, vitiligo, and tuberculoid leprosy.

Treatment

Benzathine penicillin or PAM 1.2–2.4 megaunits is usually effective. Prophylactic treatment involves raising the standard of living and hygiene, prompt treatment of diagnosed cases, and mass treatment of people in endemic areas will control the disease.

16.5   Cutaneous leishmaniasis *(oriental sore)* (figure 16.1)

This is a chronic nodular or ulcerative skin infection caused by flagellate protozoa, *Leishmania tropica* or related species. It is transmitted by tiny sand-flies, *Phlebotomus papatasii*. Leishmaniasis is a disease of the tropical and sub-tropical regions especially the Mediterranean region, the Middle East and other parts of Asia, North, West and Central Africa, and Central and South America.

Clinical features

Lesions of cutaneous leishmaniasis are usually seen on the face or other exposed parts. Following the bite of an infected sand-fly and inoculation of the protozoa into the skin, dusky nodules develop within weeks or months. These ulcers grow slowly over the months

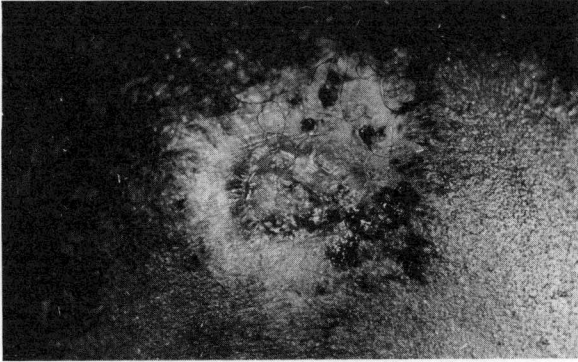

Figure 16.1   Cutaneous leishmaniasis with nodules and scarring on forehead (Courtesy: Dr J. U. Egere).

healing in parts to leave irregular scars or scaly plaques. Satellite lesions may develop.

Two other clinical forms of the disease caused by similar protozoa are:

(1) Muco-cutaneous leishmaniasis (Brazilian leishmaniasis) caused by *Leishmania braziliensis*. This affects the skin and may involve mucosa of the nose, mouth, nasopharynx and larynx. In severe cases, it may become disseminated.

(2) Visceral leishmaniasis (Kala azar) caused by *Leishmania donovani*. This affects the reticulo-endothelial system and is characterised by fever, anaemia, hepatosplenomegaly, weight loss and patchy discoloration of the skin.

Diagnosis of cutaneous leishmaniasis

This is based on the clinical picture, identification of the organisms in smears or biopsy specimens, and the demonstration in histopathological sections of granulomas with macrophages containing Leishman–Donovan bodies.

The Leishmanin or Montenegro skin test is usually positive in over 90 per cent of cases.

Treatment

In cutaneous leishmaniasis, the lesions may be injected locally with 10 per cent aqueous solution of mepacrine hydrochloride weekly until the lesions clear up.

Sodium antimony gluconate (Pentostam) 400–600 mg I.M. daily for one to two weeks or meglumine antimoniate (Glucantime) I.M. daily for 2 weeks may be given for cutaneous, muco-cutaneous or visceral leishmaniasis.

In severe cases or when the antimony injections fail, amphotericin B may be effective.

Prophylaxis

In addition to raising the standard of environmental hygiene, DDT and other insecticides can be used to reduce the population of vectors, the sand-flies.

16.6   Connective tissue diseases

These are a group of auto-immune disorders involving the skin and other organs in which fibrinoid degeneration of collagen is a common factor.

Chronic discoid lupus erythematosus (figures 16.2 and 16.3)

This is a distinctive scaling and scarring disorder characterised by symmetrical or irregular dusky erythematous plaques across the cheeks and nose (butterfly lesion), other parts of the face, scalp, neck, ears, trunk, arms or other parts of the body. The lesions are chronic, and heal irregularly leaving scars or scarring alopecia.

Female patients may or may not outnumber males. Exposure to sunlight may worsen the condition in some patients. It is rare for patients with chronic discoid lupus erythematosus to show signs of systemic disease but some laboratory tests, for example, ESR, anti-nuclear factor and rheumatoid factor may suggest systemic involvement.

Treatment Tab. chloroquine 200 mg b.d. for 4–6 weeks and then 200 mg daily is usually effective. The eyes should be examined every month to ensure that there are no corneal deposits or chloroquine retinopathy. Hydroxychloroquine (Plaquenil) 400 mg b.d. may cause milder side effects than chloroquine.

Topical corticosteroid treatment also produces good results, and should be used in conjunction with chloroquine.

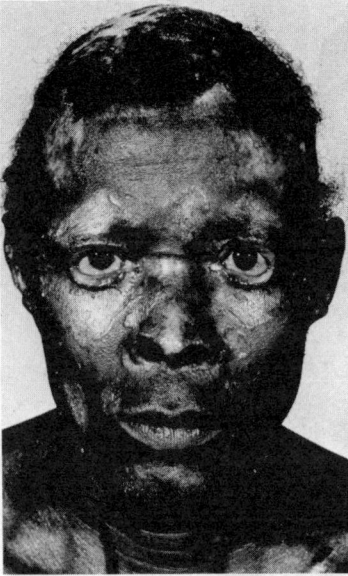

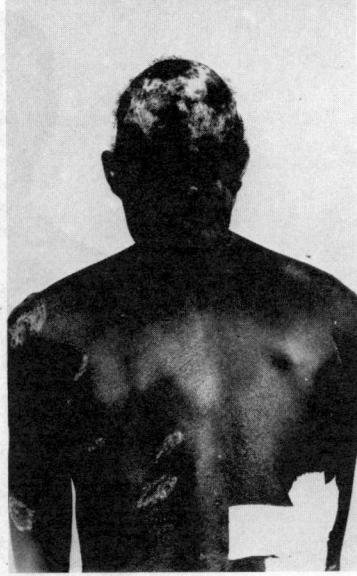

Figure 16.2   *(Left)* Chronic discoid lupus erythematosus: dusky scarring plaques on face and scalp, patchy alopecia and ectropion.

Figure 16.3   *(Right)* Chronic discoid lupus erythematosus: scarring alopecia and dusky plaques on the trunk.

Systemic lupus erythematosus (figure 16.4)

In this condition, the characteristic skin manifestations include diffuse erythema or duskiness of the face, arms and trunk, diffuse alopecia, pallor and purpura. It is however a protean disease affecting many organs – kidneys, heart and lungs, musculo-skeletal system, reticulo-endothelial system, haemopoietic system and nervous system. Females are more commonly affected than males.

The patients are usually chronically ill with fever, lassitude, pallor, mucosal erosion, muscle and joint pains. Severe systemic involvement may present as arthritis, nephritis, pericarditis, pneumonia, pleurisy, hepatosplenomegaly, lymphadenitis, epilepsy or cerebrovascular accidents.

Raynaud's phenomenon (painful spasm and coldness of the fingers) is common. The mortality rate is high from severe anaemia, renal or cardiac failure, pneumonia, vascular disorders or cerebrovascular accidents.

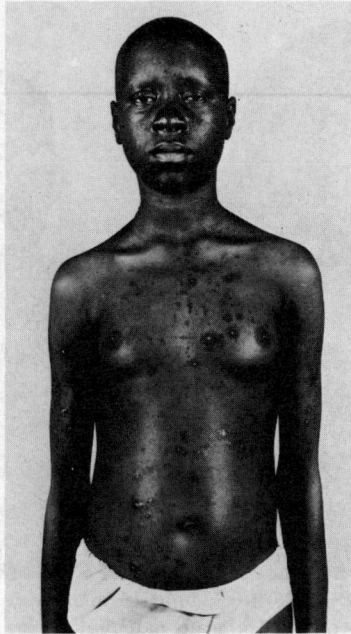

Figure 16.4   Systemic lupus erythematosus: dusky erythema on trunk and
limbs and diffuse alopecia.

Diagnosis of SLE This is based on the history, clinical features and laboratory findings. Haematological findings include high ESR, anaemia, leucopenia, thrombocytopenia and hypergamma-globulinaemia.

The LE cell phenomenon can also be demonstrated using the patient's serum or whole blood. Antinuclear factor test is strongly positive. Serological tests for syphilis and for rheumatoid factor may give false positive results.

Differential diagnosis Conditions which may be confused with SLE include rheumatoid arthritis, systemic sclerosis, Hodgkin's lymphoma, other reticuloses, and leukaemia.

Treatment Corticosteroids in high doses are useful in controlling the disease. Prednisone 60–100 mg daily until the disease is under fair control, followed by a gradual reduction until a maintenance dose of 5–15 mg daily is reached.

Patients not responding to corticosteroids may be put on immunosuppressive drugs. Azathioprine 100–200 mg daily for a long period gives good results. Other drugs include cyclophosphamide, 6-mercaptopurine and nitrogen mustard.

Blood transfusions, the control of intercurrent infection, relief of oedema in nephrotic syndrome or cardiac failure and sedation may be necessary to prolong life.

Systemic sclerosis (plate 37)

In the mild form of this condition, sometimes referred to as scleroderma, swelling and duskiness of the skin of the face and hands is followed by atrophy and binding down of the skin to underlying tissues. The mouth and nose and eyes become pinched, the fingers spindle shaped and cold, and the skin in other parts hard and bound down. Small ulcers may develop in the affected fingers.

After months or years, systemic involvement may include the oesophagus, the rest of the alimentary tract, the kidneys, heart and lungs.

Treatment Vasodilator drugs, for example, tolazoline hydrochloride (Priscol) may help to relieve the coldness of the digits. Systemic corticosteroids, calcium disodium edetate (Versenate) and chloroquine have all been found useful.

Morphoea (*localised scleroderma*)

In this condition one or more circumscribed plaques of hardened atrophic skin develop on the skin of the face, trunk or limbs. Severe lesions may involve underlying muscles and even bone.

Treatment Corticosteroids applied or injected intra-lesionally early in the disease may improve the condition.

16.7   Keloids (figures 16.5 and 16.6)

These are firm rubbery swellings of variable shapes and sizes resulting from excessive connective tissue response to skin injury or tension. Factors in keloid formation include genetic disposition, endocrine factors, and extraneous particles including keratin carried into the skin by deliberate or accidental injury.

Keloids develop on sites of scars, tattoos, vaccinations, skin decorations, ear or nose piercing, chronic inflammation, acne vulgaris, variola, varicella or other infection, surgical scars, burns or scalds.

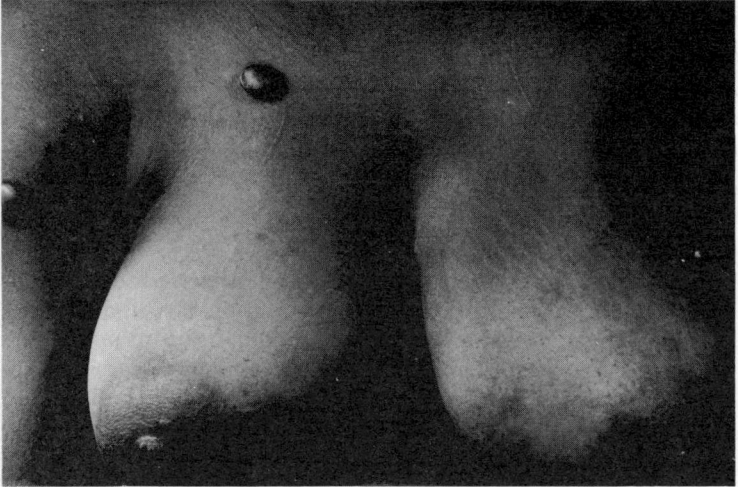

Figure 16.5   Keloids following minor injuries.

So-called spontaneous keloids develop without obvious trauma, for example, over the sternum or breasts where there is underlying strain, stretch or tension.

Rapidly growing or infected keloids may be itchy, painful or tender. Over joints, keloids may cause contractures. Small or inactive keloids are usually symptomless but most keloids are cosmetically unacceptable and some may cause disfigurement.

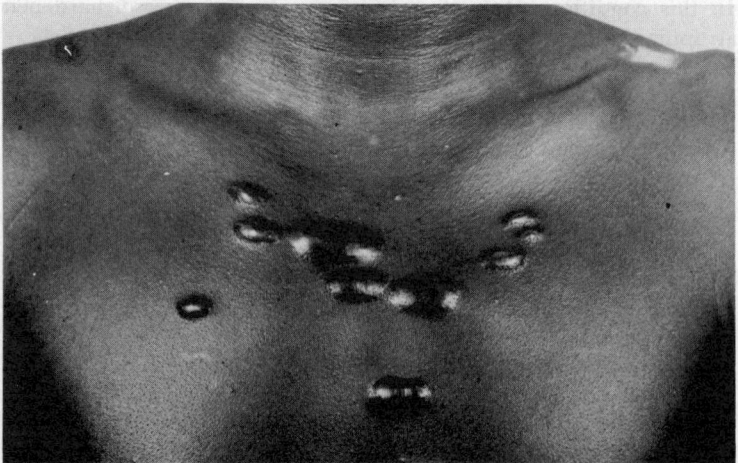

Figure 16.6   Keloids following acne vulgaris.

Treatment

Some keloids regress spontaneously even if incompletely, and there-fore need no treatment.

Some young keloids regress in response to topical application of corticosteroid sprays, creams or ointments or the intra-lesional injec-tion of corticosteroids. Many keloids have the tendency to recur and increase in size after excision. Considering the high rate of recurrence after excision, only keloids which are large or unsightly should be excised and preferably where there are facilities for pre-operative and post-operative radiotherapy.

16.8   **Ichthyosis** *('fish skin')* (figure 16.7)

In this condition the skin is covered all over with rough dry scales, sparing mainly the flexures. Ichthyosis is an inherited disorder (autosomal dominant gene), appears in infancy or early childhood, and persists throughout life with some periods of slight spontaneous improvement. It is a disorder of the normal process of keratinisation.

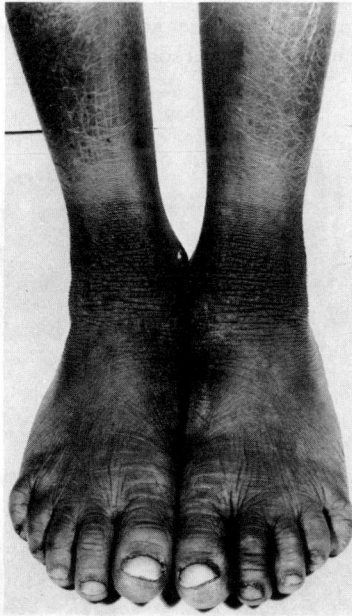

Figure 16.7   Ichthyosis.

The normal rate of removal of the horny layer is reduced and the keratin formed is therefore heaped up.

Treatment is difficult and often disappointing. Ointments containing salicylic acid 3 per cent in emulsifying ointment sometimes help. Large doses of vitamin A by mouth over a period of months may improve some cases. Cosmetically acceptable creams should be given to tone down the dryness and roughness of the skin, for example, urea 10 per cent in a water-miscible base.

16.9 **Keratoderma of the palms and soles** (figures 16.8–16.10)

In this condition, the palms and soles are dusky, thick and scaly, the disorder sometimes extending to the sides of the hands and feet, to the wrists and ankles and even up the forearms and lower legs.

It is usually inherited (autosomal dominant gene), and may appear in childhood or late in life. Painful fissures may develop and walking and the use of the hands may be impaired. Sometimes the condition may develop later in life without any trace of family history.

Salicylic acid ointment and other keratolytic applications may help to soften the thickened palms and soles.

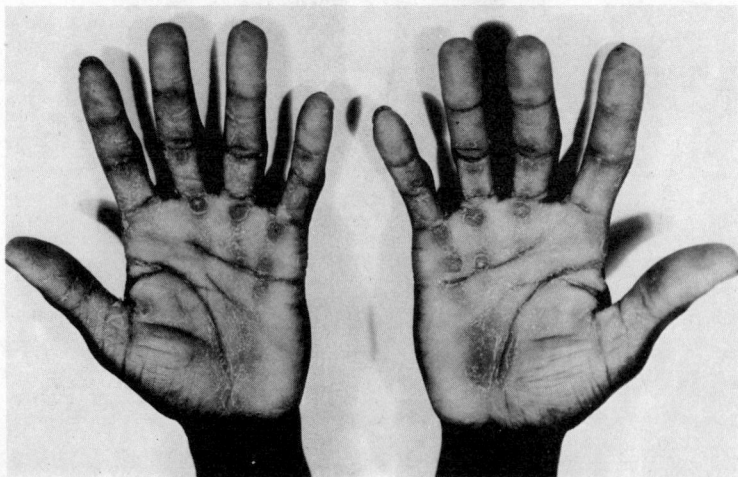

Figure 16.8   Keratoderma with palmar hyperkeratosis.

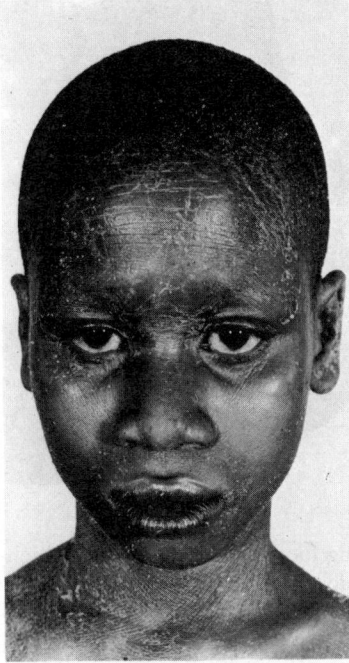

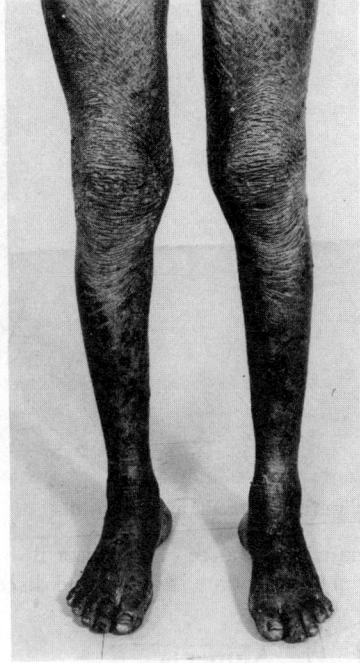

Figure 16.9   *(Left)* Chronic erythroderma with generalised exfoliation.

Figure 16.10   *(Right)* Chronic erythroderma with generalised exfoliation.

16.10   **Pressure hyperkeratosis of the palms and soles**
(figure 16.11)

Localised callosities of the soles develop commonly in people wearing hard or ill-fitting footwear. The balls of the feet and the heels are the common starting points, pressure over the metatarsal heads and the calcaneum being the cause of the constant friction. The callosities may extend to involve other areas of the soles. Painful fissures may develop and make walking difficult.

Callosities (corns) over the toes and between the toes may also impair walking. They are also due to constant friction between bony points and ill-fitting footwear.

Treatment

Paring of callosities, application of keratolytic agents, wearing of corn

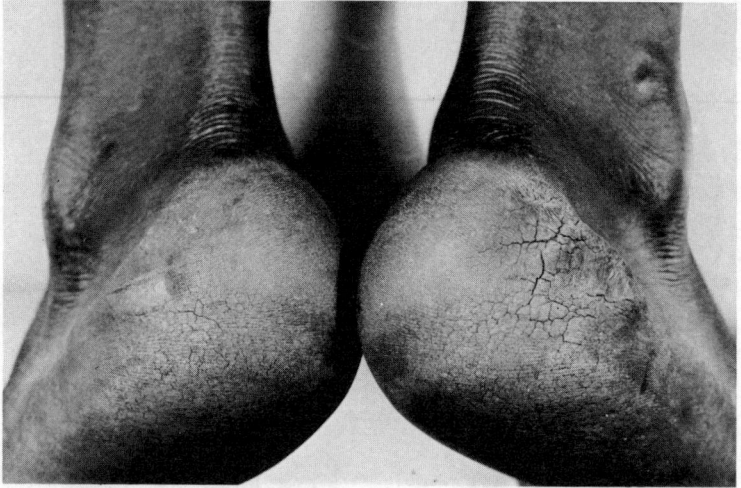

Figure 16.11   Plantar callosities.

pads, avoidance of closed or ill-fitting footwear are measures which help to alleviate the pain and discomfort.

16.11   Alopecia

Loss of hair worries men and women alike. A proper understanding of each of the various types of alopecia is necessary to be able to offer the correct advice to the sufferer.

Male pattern baldness

This is usually inherited, starts with recession in the temples, and then encroaches on the vertex. In severe cases the baldness ends up leaving a horse-shoe shaped band of hair covering the back of the scalp and extending forwards above the ears. The vertex is smooth and shiny. It may start in the early twenties and be fully developed in the thirties or forties.

If seborrhoea capitis (dandruff) coexists or appears to be in the background, treating the seborrhoea may slow down the pace of development of alopecia.

Traumatic alopecia in women

Frequent plaiting of the hair or other energetic hair care procedures may produce alopecia starting along the hair line and progressing towards the vertex. Detecting the form of trauma and eliminating or minimising it can improve cases of traumatic alopecia.

Trichotillomania (plate 38)

A compulsive pulling of the hair due to psychological upset may produce a patchy alopecia over a variable portion of the scalp. For trichotillomania, unravelling and removing the underlying psychological disturbance must be achieved before the hair can regrow.

Alopecia areata (figure 16.12 and plate 39)

In this condition, there is a sudden appearance of one or more circular patches of hair loss on the scalp. The skin is shiny and looks and feels healthy. The bald patches may extend and then become static. Spontaneous and complete regrowth of hair usually takes place after many months, but some cases may progress to alopecia totalis and may be complicated by nail deformities and vitiligo. The cause is unknown, but emotional stress can be traced in a number of patients.

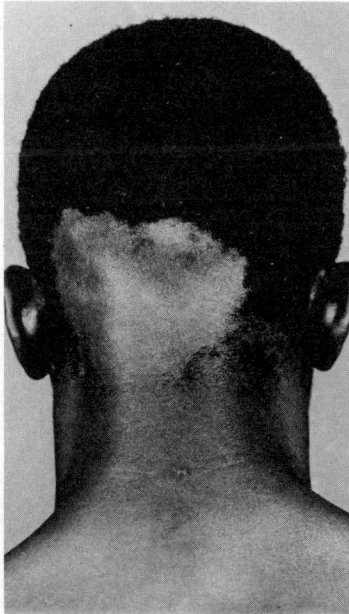

Figure 16.12   Alopecia areata: symptomless smooth punched-out hair loss.

Genetic, endocrine and immunological factors may also operate in alopecia areata.

Treatment Reassurance about a good prognosis and the gentle application of rubifacient or other scalp creams or lotions will usually help the patient await the regrowth of hair.

In chronic or recurrent alopecia areata or in alopecia totalis intra-lesional injections of corticosteroids may help to regrow the hair. If alopecia totalis becomes permanent, a wig may be supplied and the patient assisted psychologically to adjust.

Symptomatic alopecia

Diffuse hair loss may follow febrile illness or other constitutional diseases or constitutional upsets such as childbirth, major surgery, endocrine diseases, anaemia, nutritional deficiency, reticuloses or neoplasms. Management of these types would depend on diagnosing correctly the underlying disease or disorder, and giving appropriate treatment.

17 Skin Markers of Systemic Diseases

The skin is in intimate physical contact with underlying tissues, and in intimate functional contact with other organs in the body. It acts as a window not only on the underlying structures, but also on near or distant internal organs.

The skin's body-guard functions include sensing and mirroring pathological changes in underlying structures and internal organs. The skin signals its observations by displaying non-specific symptoms such as pruritus, pricking or pain; by displaying non-specific primary and/or secondary skin lesions; or by displaying specific visible and palpable pathology identical with, similar to or pathognomonic of pathological changes in the diseased internal organ.

The pruritus of diabetes mellitus, obstructive jaundice and the lymphomas; the pain of herpes zoster and tabes dorsalis; the anaesthesia of neural leprosy and syringomyelia; the central cyanosis of Fallot's tetralogy and veno-arterial shunts; the hyperpigmentation of Addison's disease are all outward visible signs of underlying diseased organs.

The Koplik's spots of measles, the fixed erythema of lupus erythematosus, the nodules of erythema nodosum, the xanthomata of hyperlipaemia, the bullae of porphyria, the telangiectasia of liver disease, the hirsutism of Cushing's syndrome, the koilonychia of severe iron deficiency anaemia, all reflect systemic disorders.

The hidden secrets of neoplasms of internal organs are sometimes betrayed by the skin. The flushing attacks in malignant argentaffinoma (carcinoid syndrome), the buccal mucosal pigmented macules in intestinal polyposis (Peutz-Jegher's syndrome) and the diffuse melanosis of malignant melanoma are examples of skin markers of internal neoplasms.

Skin diseases with internal manifestations include atopic eczema, psoriasis, neurofibromatosis, rosacea, urticaria pigmentosa and incontinentia pigmenti.

The major cutaneous symptoms and pigmentary changes and the important systemic diseases with which they are associated will be described. Then the distinctive primary and/or secondary skin lesions and the related systemic diseases will be listed in tabular form. The skin markers of internal malignancy and the internal manifestations of cutaneous disorders will similarly be presented in tabular form.

17.1 **Pruritus** (*(itching)*)

Itching is by far the commonest symptom of skin diseases. Generalised itching is also the commonest cutaneous symptom associated with internal diseases.

Diabetes mellitus

In diabetes mellitus, the skin is dry because of a decrease in the surface lipid and a decrease in water-holding capacity of the horny layer of the epidermis. Superficial fissuring and fine scaling result, and itching is due to a combination of all these factors. Ano-genital itching in diabetic patients especially women may be due additionally to ano-genital candidiasis (moniliasis). Other common endocrine and metabolic diseases in which itching may be marked include myxoedema, hyperthyroidism, and gout.

Liver diseases

In biliary obstruction, biliary cirrhosis, hepatocellular jaundice or post-hepatic jaundice, itching is due to increase in bile salts in the system. Gall-stones and carcinoma of the pancreas, colon or stomach obstructing the biliary ducts will also cause severe itching.

Renal diseases

In uraemia, the high blood urea may be reflected on the skin as diffuse greyish pigmentation and this may be associated with moderate or severe itching.

Anaemia

In severe iron deficiency anaemia, megaloblastic anaemia and sickle cell anaemia, there may be mild or moderate itching. Polycythaemia also causes marked itching.

Leukaemia

In both myelocytic and lymphocytic leukaemia, itching is a marked feature, and may precede changes in blood picture by months or even years.

Diseases of the reticulo-endothelial system

In Hodgkin's lymphoma, non-Hodgkin lymphomas, lymphosarcoma, reticulum cell sarcoma, severe itching may precede the disease by many months or even years. In mycosis fungoides and Sezary's syndrome, severe itching accompanies the eczematous and infiltrative stages while the tumours in mycosis fungoides develop years later.

Infestations

Helminthic infestations, filarial infestations and tropical eosinophilia induce moderate to severe itching.

Allergic and auto-immune diseases

Urticaria, dermographism, systemic lupus erythematosus and dermatomyositis cause intense pruritus.

Neuropsychiatric diseases

Neurological syphilis, anxiety and obsessional neurosis are all associated with itching.

Pregnancy

Itching is usual in the third trimester and is probably hormonal in origin. Glycosuria and candidiasis may be additional causes.

17.2 Burning, pricking, pain and anaesthesia

Herpes zoster

The tense vesicles of herpes zoster may be preceded by burning or pain in the cutaneous distribution of the nerve infected by the virus. Pain accompanies the eruption of herpes zoster throughout, and post-herpetic neuralgia persists in some cases long after healing of the herpetic lesions. Herpes zoster may be associated with Hodgkin's and non-Hodgkin lymphomas, leukaemia, and visceral carcinoma.

Tabes dorsalis

The shooting or stabbing pains down the trunk and legs or round the chest accompanied by pins and needles or numbness in the feet are characteristic of tertiary syphilis in which there is atrophy of the posterior roots of the spinal nerves and of the posterior columns of the spinal cord up to the nuclei gracilis and cuneatus.

Leprosy

Patches of anaesthesia may precede by many months, the hypopig-mented patches of leprosy in the same areas.

Syringomyelia

Loss of pain and temperature sensations in the fingers, with preserva-tion of tactile sensation is an early manifestation of syringomyelia in which there is cavitation surrounded by gliosis in the spinal cord starting in the upper thoracic or lower cervical region.

17.3 Pigmentary changes

These show principally, alterations in the skin colour.

Cyanosis

This is a bluish or purplish tinge due to an excess of reduced haemoglobin resulting from impaired oxygenation or circulation of blood. Central cyanosis is seen in heart diseases, for example, congen-ital heart diseases with veno-arterial shunts, and respiratory diseases, for example, emphysema, pulmonary oedema, and pneumonia. It is also seen in polycythaemia vera.

Peripheral cyanosis is seen in the extremities when the circulation is sluggish and there is an excessive abstraction of oxygen from the

A combination of central cyanosis and peripheral cyanosis is seen in congestive cardiac failure.

Pallor

This occurs in anaemia (the inverted lower lid gives a good indica-tion). It is also seen in fainting and in severe nausea and vomiting.

Jaundice

A yellowish colour of the skin and mucous membranes due to excess of bilirubin in the plasma and tissue fluids occurs in the various types of jaundice: pre-hepatic or haemolytic, hepatic and post-hepatic or obstructive.

Hyperpigmentation

Addison's disease There is generalised hyperpigmentation giving a dark brown to almost black colour to the skin especially the exposed parts, the pressure areas, the axillae, areola and nipples of the breasts and the external genitalia. The creases of the palms and soles and the buccal mucosa are all hyperpigmented. This condition is due to adrenocortical hormone deficiency resulting from atrophy of the adrenal glands or their destruction by disease, for example, tuberculosis.

Haemochromatosis (bronze diabetes) Dark brown or slaty-grey hyperpigmentation may result from excessive deposition of iron in the liver.

Metallic poisoning Chronic arsenic poisoning may produce widespread mottled hyperpigmentation especially of the covered parts.

Silver poisoning (argyria) – a slaty-grey hyperpigmentation is produced by deposition of silver in the skin.

Acanthosis nigricans Hyperpigmentation with verrucose or papillomatous lesions in the axillae and groins is associated in about 50 per cent of cases with carcinoma of the stomach or other organs.

Carotenaemia Yellowish coloration of the skin (most evident on the palms) is caused by excessive ingestion of carrots or other carotene-containing yellow vegetables.

Localised hyperpigmentation This is seen in hyperthyroidism, pellagra, rheumatoid arthritis and pregnancy.

Depigmentation

Phenylketonuria is associated with epilepsy and mental deficiency.
 Alkaptonuria is associated with arthropathy.
 Vitiligo may be associated with diffuse or systemic scleroderma, clinical or latent diabetes mellitus, Addison's pernicious anaemia, or thyrotoxicosis.

Purpura

Escape of blood from a vessel into the skin, mucosae or joints may be due to platelet disorders (thrombocytopenia) or vascular abnormalities. Small petechiae or purpuric spots do not disappear on pressure, neither do large ecchymoses. Purpura may be idiopathic but may also be an indication of leukaemia, amyloidosis, Cushing's disease, bacterial endocarditis, uraemia, meningococcal meningitis, and viral and rickettsial diseases.

Drugs which can cause toxic purpura include penicillin, sulphonamides, salicylates and barbiturates.

17.4   Distinctive lesions

Some ordinary skin lesions are associated with systemic diseases and should therefore not be taken in isolation. Thorough and systematic examination should always be conducted however simple the skin lesion may look.

Table 17.1   Skin Lesions Associated with Systemic Diseases

Lesion	Systemic Diseases
Acneiform papules	Pituitary, adrenal, ovarian or testicular disorders. Drugs: bromides, iodides, corticosteroids or androgens.
Chronic ulcers	Sickle cell anaemia, spherocytosis, ulcerative colitis.
Erythema multiforme	Rheumatic fever, typhoid fever, viral infections, deep fungal infections, malaria, connective tissue diseases, polycythaemia, drug eruptions.
Erythema nodosum	Streptococcal infections, tuberculosis, leprosy, sarcoidosis, leukaemia, deep fungal infections, ulcerative colitis. Drugs: sulphonamides, diaminodiphenylsulphone, bromides, iodides.
Juxta-articular nodes	Rheumatoid arthritis, syphilis, yaws, pinta.

Table 17.1 (*continued*)

Lesion	Systemic Diseases
Macules	Typhoid fever (rose spots), measles, infectious mononucleosis.
Pustules	Diabetes mellitus, reticuloses.
Telangiectasia	Liver cirrhosis, leukaemia and other blood dyscrasias, endocrine disorders.
Urticaria	Rheumatic fever, systemic lupus erythematosus, serum hepatitis, Hodgkin's lymphoma.
Vesicles/bullae	Febrile illnesses, lymphomas, reticuloses, porphyria, pemphigoid, dermatitis herpetiformis, epidermolysis bullosa.
Xanthomata	Hyperlipaemia

Table 17.2   Other Cutaneous Manifestations Associated with Systemic Diseases

Manifestations	Systemic Diseases
Adenoma sebaceum	Tuberose sclerosis.
Candidiasis	Diabetes mellitus, prolonged wide-spectrum antibiotic therapy, prolonged systemic corticosteroid therapy.
Dermatitis artefacta	Emotional tension, malingering
Eczema/dermatitis	Hodgkin's and non-Hodgkin lymphomas, mycosis fungoides, Sezary's syndrome, leukaemia, drug eruptions.
Gingival bleeding	Scurvy (vitamin C deficiency)
Gingival hypertrophy	Prolonged phenytoin sodium therapy, leukaemia.
Hippocratic nails	Cyanotic congenital heart diseases, chronic lung diseases, carcinoma of the lungs.

Table 17.2 (*continued*)

Manifestations	Systemic Diseases
Hirsutism	Cushing's syndrome, ovarian tumours, overdose with ACTH
Hyperhirosis (generalised)	Tuberculosis, hyperthyroidism.
Hyperhidrosis (localised)	Emotional stress.
Hypertrichosis	Porphyria.
Koilonychia	Severe iron deficiency anaemia.
Macroglossia	Systemic amyloidosis.
Magenta tongue	Riboflavine deficiency.
Mouth ulcers	Aphthous stomatitis, toxic erythema multiforme, pemphigus, secondary syphilis.
Nail biting	Anxiety, repressed emotion.
Nail pigmentation	Prolonged widespectrum antibiotic therapy, heavy metal poisoning, for example, silver.
Neurotic excoriations	Nervousness, anxiety.
Angular cheilitis or perleche	Vitamin B deficiency, severe iron-deficiency anaemia, candidiasis.
Pale atrophic tongue	Addison's pernicious anaemia.
Parasitophobia	Psychoneurosis, psychosis.
Rhagades	Congenital syphilis.
Neurodermatitis	Endocrine disorders (premenstrual, menopausal), emotional stress.

17.5   Skin markers of internal malignancy

The skin can mirror the presence of internal cancer in a number of ways. Sometimes these skin manifestations accompany the manifest disease. At other times, they helpfully appear before the cancer is manifest and can therefore help in deciding on early treatment of the cancer.

The mechanisms of these cutaneous reflections of internal cancer are not always definite. Auto-allergic reactions and hormonal reactions are among the possible mechanisms.

Table 17.3   Cutaneous Manifestations of Internal Malignancy

Manifestation	Associated internal malignancy
Generalised pruritus	Hodgkin's and non-Hodgkin lymphomas, leukaemia, multiple myelomatosis, polycythaemia vera, carcinoma of the liver, gastrointestinal tract, breast or ovary.
Acanthosis nigricans	Carcinoma of the gastrointestinal tract, breast, lungs or other viscera.
Amyloidosis	Multiple myelomatosis.
Dermatomyositis	Carcinoma of the breast or ovary, sarcoma, reticulo-endothelial neoplasms.
Diffuse melanosis	Malignant melanoma, pituitary tumours producing melanocyte-stimulating hormones (MSH), and carcinoma of the adrenal gland.
Erythema multiforme	Leukaemia, carcinoma of the thyroid, lungs and other viscera.
Erythema nodosum	Leukaemia, Hodgkin's lymphoma, secondary carcinomatous deposits.
Erythroderma	Hodgkin's lymphoma, leukaemia, Sezary's syndrome.
Exfoliative dermatitis	Leukaemia, mycosis fungoides, Sezary's syndrome.
Flushing attacks	Malignant argentaffinoma.
Hyperkeratosis (palms and soles)	Hodgkin's lymphoma, leukaemia, Sezary's syndrome.
Ichthyosis (acquired)	Hodgkin's lymphoma, reticuloses.

Table 17.3 (*continued*)

Manifestation	Associated internal malignancy
Purpura	Leukaemia, Hodgkin's lymphoma, multiple myelomatosis.
Urticaria	Hodgkin's and non-Hodgkin lymphomas, leukaemia, carcinoma of the gastro-intestinal tract, hydatidiform mole.

Table 17.4   Internal Manifestations of Skin Diseases

Manifestations/Syndromes	Associated Skin Disease
Arthritis involving the small joints	Psoriasis.
Bone and teeth deformities, epilepsy, mental deficiency	Incontinentia pigmenti.
Bronchial asthma, hay fever, migraine, cataracts	Atopic eczema.
Eye disorders (blepharitis, keratoconjunctivitis).	Rosacea.
Mastocytosis involving lymph node, bone, liver and thymus gland	Urticaria pigmentosa.
Retinal angioid streaks, peripheral vascular disorders, gastrointestinal haemorrhage and mental changes	Pseudoxanthoma elasticum.
Spinal and cranial nerve tumours, deafness, epilepsy, paralysis and sensory disorders.	Multiple neurofibromatosis.

18 Sexually Transmitted Diseases

The association between skin diseases and sexually transmitted diseases stems from the manifestations on the skin and mucous membranes of many sexually transmitted diseases. Syphilis was the STD primarily responsible for this association. It has cutaneous manifestations in its primary, secondary and tertiary states.

Sexually transmitted diseases have been with the human race for a long time. They are usually spread by heterosexual or homosexual contact. Their effects may be localised to the region of contact, or may become spread to distant organs.

STD is usually blamed on the other person. In the early days of syphilis in Europe, it was called 'French disease', 'Spanish disease' or 'Italian disease' by others. In developing countries men fancifully call all STD 'women's disease'.

18.1 Classification of STD

Sexually transmitted diseases may be grouped into major and minor groups.

Major group

These have high prevalence, genital discharge or genital or skin swellings or ulcers, and systemic involvement.

(1) Syphilis
(2) Gonorrhoea
(3) Non-specific urethritis (non-gonoccal urethritis)
(4) Chancroid
(5) Granuloma inguinale
(6) Lymphogranuloma venereum

Minor group

These have genital discharge or mild local genital lesions.

(1) Trichomonal infection
(2) Candida infection
(3) Genital herpes

  (4) Genital warts (condyloma acuminata)
  (5) Molluscum contagiosum
  (6) Scabies
  (7) Pediculosis pubis

18.2   Syphilis

This is the STD with the greatest potential for systemic spread to involve other organs. History has it that Christopher Columbus' men imported it from the New World (America) to Europe and then with the subsequent spread of European civilisation went 'syphilisation'. It is caused by the spirochaete *Treponema pallidum* and is normally limited to man.

Natural history

Following sexual exposure and subsequent infection, the natural history of the disease is in three main stages.

Primary stage (hard chancre) (figure 18.1) At the site of entry into the body (external genitalia in heterosexuals, anus in homosexuals or lips in perverts) the organisms multiply and a firm papule is formed within a few weeks. This papule may ulcerate to produce the painless primary syphilitic ulcer which may 'heal' quite early. *Treponema pallidum* can be isolated from the ulcers. Lymphatic and blood stream spread may begin even at this early stage.

Secondary stage From one to two months later, a varied picture of lesions showing the systemic nature of the disease may appear on various parts of the body. These lesions include widespread dusky maculo-papules on the face, neck, trunk and hands and feet, erosions on the mucosa of the mouth, moist wart-like papules (condylomata lata) in the ano-genital region, and lymph node enlargement. There may also be alopecia, periostitis and signs of meningeal involvement. *Treponema pallidum* is abundant in secondary lesions. These lesions are therefore highly infectious. Serological tests are positive at this stage.

Tertiary stage Systemic spread of the disease continues, and lesions develop after months or years in the affected organs. Degenerative changes occur in the brain and spinal cord and in the cardiovascular system, while granulomatous lesions develop in the skin (gummata),

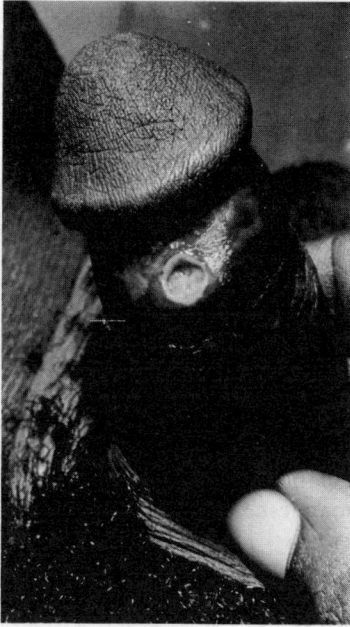

Figure 18.1 Primary chancre.

bone and liver. Tertiary lesions are produced mainly by immunological reactions to *Treponema pallidum*.

Congenital syphilis

During pregnancy, *Treponema pallidum* in an infected woman passes through the placenta to infect the foetus. The manifestations of syphilis in the baby will depend on the degree of damage to developing organs. At birth, the baby may be covered with bullae, or these bullae may develop some weeks or months later. The mucous membrane of the mouth, nose and eyes may also be infected. Like the lesions of secondary syphilis, all these lesions are highly infectious.

Other stigmata of congenital syphilis which may appear in later childhood include keratitis, saddle nose, jaw and teeth deformities, nerve deafness, sabre tibia.

Diagnosis of syphilis

In all cases, a history of sexual exposure should be sought carefully and obtained. This is vital for the tracing and treatment of sexual contacts.

Primary stage
 (1) Nodules or chancres on the external genitalia, anus or lips.
 (2) Microscopic examination for *Treponema pallidum* in smears or scrapings from chancres (dark field examinations).
 (3) Serological tests are seldom positive.

Secondary stage
 (1) The clinical picture of cutaneous and mucosal lesions. There may also be lymphadenitis and alopecia.
 (2) Microscopic examination of smears from lesions for *Treponema pallidum* (dark field examination).
 (3) Serological tests which are usually positive include:
    (a) VDRL test – (venereal disease research laboratory). This is a flocculation test.
    (b) Wasserman test.
    (c) Kahn test.
    (d) Treponemal immobilisation test.
    (e) Fluorescent treponemal antibody absorption test (FTA–ABS).

Tertiary stage
 (1) The clinical picture
    (a) Gummata on skin.
    (b) Aortic valve incompetence or aortic aneurysm.
    (c) Degenerative changes in spinal cord, meninges or cerebrum. Clinical picture of tabes dorsalis or general paresis of the insane.
 (2) Serological tests.
 (3) Cerebrospinal fluid examination: cells, protein, Lange curve, complement fixation test, VDRL test.

Treatment of syphilis

Penicillin remains a very effective antibiotic in the treatment of syphilis. It exerts its effect on the slowly dividing treponema. In early stages of infection (under 1 year) procaine penicillin 1.2 megaunits I.M. daily for 2 weeks or benzathine penicillin 2.4 megaunits I.M. weekly for 2 weeks.

In late stages (over 1 year) procaine penicillin treatment should be continued for 3–4 weeks, or benzathine penicillin 2.4 megaunits may be given 3 times weekly for 2 weeks. Probenecid 1 g orally daily during treatment with high doses of penicillin.

In patients with hypersensitivity to penicillin, 1g erythromycin or tetracycline (except in pregnancy) may be given daily for 2–4 weeks.

Follow-up tests including serological tests should be continued for 1–2 years.

In congenital syphilis, because of the inability of benzathine penicillin to enter the CSF readily, procane penicillin 600,000 units daily for 10–14 days is preferable.

18.3 Gonorrhoea

This is the STD with the greatest reported incidence world wide and the one with the steepest rising graph in many countries.

It is caused by *Neisseria gonorrhoeae* – Gram-negative intracellular diplococci usually seen within pus cells in smears from infected patients.

Natural history

Following sexual exposure, infection is established in the mucous membrane and acute suppuration occurs. Clinical manifestations vary in both sexes.

Males In males, within a few days to one week of exposure, burning or pain on urination and urethritis with whitish or yellowish pus from the urethra characterise the acute infection. In homosexuals and oral sex perverts, acute infections may manifest as proctitis and pharyngitis or tonsillitis respectively. The conjunctiva may also become infected accidentally.

Sub-acute or chronic extension of urethritis may lead to posterior urethritis, peri-urethral abscess, cystitis, prostatitis, seminal vesiculitis and epididymitis or epididymo-orchitis.

Urethral stricture is the most severe local complication of gonorhoea in males. It causes complications backwards to involve the prostate, urinary bladder, ureters and kidneys.

Blood stream spread of *Neisseria gonorrhoeae* may also lead to periostitis, arthritis, conjunctivitis, endocarditis or meningitis.

Females Acute infection in females tends to cause less pain and discomfort than in males but infection and suppuration of various mucous membranes occurs. Vaginitis, cervicitis, urethritis, proctitis and salpingitis are the characteristic features. Bartholinitis may also develop. In oral sex perverts, pharyngitis and tonsillitis may also occur.

Chronic infection may lead to cystitis, salpingo-oophoritis, pyosalpinx, pelvic inflammatory disease, tubal fibrosis and occlusion and infertility. As in males, blood stream spread of infection may lead to periostitis, arthritis, conjunctivitis, endocarditis and meningitis.

At birth, babies of infected mothers may develop gonococcal ophthalmia neonatorum due to infection of the eyes during passage through the birth canal.

Diagnosis of gonorrhoea

As in syphilis, a history of sexual exposure is vital for the tracing and treatment of sexual contacts.

(1) Smears from urethra, cervix, anus, rectum or pharynx should be examined microscopically for Gram-negative intracellular diplococci within pus cells.
(2) Culture for *Neisseria gonorrhoeae* using selective media.
(3) Antibiotic sensitivity tests for isolated microorganisms.
(4) Two-glass urine test for haze and threads. Urine passed into two glasses will show haze and threads in the first glass if only the anterior urethra is affected (early cases), but will show haze and threads in both glasses if the posterior urethra is also affected (late cases).
(5) Serological tests for syphilis.

Treatment

For patients not allergic to it, procaine penicillin remains a cheap and effective antibiotic. The rising prevalence of penicillin-resistant strains of *Neisseria gonorrhoeae* however calls for more and more use of the more expensive antibiotics. Single dose treatment where possible should be preferred.

2.4   megaunits of procaine penicillin I.M. (1.2 megaunits into each buttock).
2.4   megaunits of benzathine penicillin (I.M.)
Ampicillin 2–3 g stat with 2 g of probenecid to delay excertion.

In patients with penicillin hypersensitivity or infected with penicillin-resistant strains:

2 g of spectinomycin hydrochloride (I.M.) stat
Tetracycline 2 g orally stat
Kanamycin 2 g orally stat

Cephaloridine 2 g orally stat
Co-trimoxazole (Septrin) 2 g b.d. for 2 days

Spaced treatment, daily with procaine penicillin for one week or twice weekly with Penadur (long-acting penicillin) or with tetracycline or other orally administered antibiotics may be used to maintain a high enough serum level for long enough to eliminate the organisms.

Follow-up Whether the treatment is single dose or spaced, follow-up examinations for 1–4 weeks are essential to monitor cure or progress.

18.4   Non-specific urethritis

STD with genital discharge not due to *Neisseria gonorrhoeae* shows a high and rising prevalence in many parts of the world. The causal organisms are various: *Chlamydia trachomatis*, anaerobic organisms, staphylococci, *Trichomonas vaginalis*, etc.

Following sexual exposure, symptoms of NSU develop more slowly than in gonococcal urethritis but infection affects practically the same organs.

Reiter's syndrome is a complication of urethritis involving acute or chronic arthritis, conjunctivitis and sometimes endocarditis.

In males, urethritis, proctitis, prostatitis, periostitis, urethritis and endocarditis and conjunctivitis may develop. In females, vaginitis, cervicitis, proctitis and periostitis, arthritis, and endocarditis and conjunctivitis may develop.

Diagnosis of NSU

(1) A history of exposure.
(2) Microscopy, culture and antibiotic sensitivity tests on secretions.
(3) Serological tests for syphilis, for exclusion.

Treatment of NSU

This should depend on the result of antibiotic sensitivity tests. Tetracycline in various dosage schedules has been found effective in the treatment of NSU.

One gram daily (in divided doses) for 2–3 weeks can be accepted as a safe regime. Failure rate may be high and re-treatment necessary. Follow-up examinations to monitor progress should always be conducted for up to 12 months if possible.

18.5   Chancroid, granuloma inguinale and lymphogranuloma venereum

These three STDs are commoner in the tropics and sub-tropics than in the temperate regions. They present with ulcers or swellings on the skin or genital mucous membranes rather than with urethral discharge.

Chancroid (figure 18.2)

This STD is caused by *Haemophilus ducreyi*, Gram-negative bacteria which enter the body through genital skin or mucous membrane. Painful ulcers (soft sores) develop at the site of entry, and the infection spreads to regional lymph nodes which soon suppurate and develop sinuses. The ulcers may ultimately heal with deep scarring.

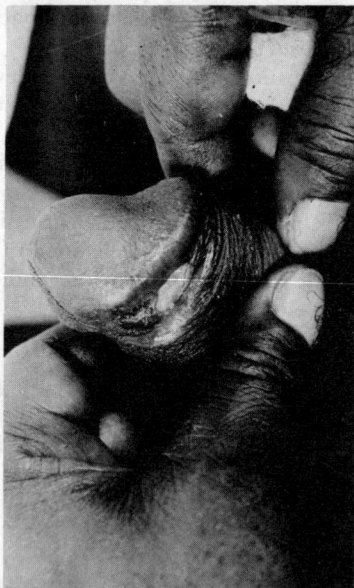

Figure 18.2   Chancroid.

Diagnosis

   (1) Clinical picture of genital ulcers and suppurating or ulcerating regional lymph nodes.

   (2) Isolation of *Haemophilus ducreyi* from smears or scrapings from ulcers or lymph nodes.

   (3) Ito skin test with dmelcos is usually positive.
   (4) Serological test for syphilis, in case both conditions co-exist.

Treatment Sulphonamides alone or in combination with antibiotics are often effective.

Short-acting sulphonamides, for example, sulphadimidine or sulphathiazole 2 g daily (in divided doses) for 2 weeks.
Long-acting sulphonamides, for example, co-trimoxazole (Septrin) 2 g daily (in divided doses) for 2 weeks.
Tetracycline 1 g daily (in divided doses) for 2 weeks.
Streptomycin 1 g (I.M.) daily for 2 weeks.

When lesions are secondarily infected with anaerobic organisms, penicillin or clindamycin may be helpful.

Granuloma inguinale (plate 40)

This STD is caused by *Donovania granulomatis*, Gram-negative bacteria which enter the body through genital skin. Following sexual exposure, slowly growing granulomatous swellings develop on the genitalia and spread to the groins and perineum. They later break down and ulcerate, the ulcers running a more chronic course than those of chancroid. Deep scarring follows subsequent healing.

Diagnosis
   (1) Clinical picture of granulomatous ulcers.
   (2) Isolation of bacteria from lesions.
   (3) Serological tests for syphilis, in case both conditions co-exist.

Treatment Streptomycin and tetracycline in adequate dosage are usually effective. Treatment should be for 2–3 weeks.
   Ampicillin 1 g daily (in divided doses) or erythromycin 1 g daily (in divided doses) for 2–3 weeks.

Chloramphenicol may be useful as a support for any of the other treatment regimes but its use is limited by its toxicity to the haemopoeitic system.

Lymphogranuloma venereum

This STD is caused by *Chlamydia trachomatis* which are difficult to isolate except in research centres.
   Following sexual exposure, infection of the genital skin and mucosa

occur. There may be non-specific (non-gonococcal) urethritis. Lymphatic spread occurs to regional lymph nodes in the genitalia, perineum, rectum and groins. These lymph nodes enlarge chronically. There may also be constitutional upset such as anorexia, fever, headache and myalgia. LGV swellings do not usually ulcerate.

Diagnosis
  (1) Clinical picture of lymphadenitis.
  (2) Isolation of *Chlamydia* from lymph nodes.
  (3) Lygranum skin test is positive.
  (4) Serological tests for syphilis, in case both conditions co-exist.

Treatment Sulphonamides, tetracycline, erythromycin and oleandomycin in adequate doses are effective against LGV.

18.6   Trichomonal infection

This STD is caused by *Trichomonas vaginalis*, a pear-shaped flagellate protozoon. Following sexual exposure, urethral or vaginal discharge may occur in 1–4 weeks.

The condition is more common in females than in males. Vaginal discharge may be scanty initially but may then become copious, frothy, whitish, yellowish or greenish later. Pruritus is common and the labia may be reddish or sore due to scratching. There is associated dysuria from involvement of the urethra and bladder.

In males, urethritis with urethral discharge and dysuria and involvement of the glans penis are the usual features.

Diagnosis
  (1) Clinical picture of urethral or vaginal discharge and local soreness.
  (2) Demonstration in fresh smears on a microscope slide of motile flagellate, *Trichomonas vaginalis*.
  (3) Urine microscopy for *Trichomonas* and other organisms.
  (4) Microscopy and culture for concomitant *Neisseria gonorrhoeae* and other organisms.
  (5) Serological tests for syphilis, in case both conditions co-exist.

Treatment

Metronidazole (Flagyl) is the specific drug for trichomoniasis. Dose 200 mg t.i.d. for 10 days.

Follow-up examinations to monitor progress are essential.

18.7 Candidiasis

This STD is caused by *Candida albicans*, a Gram-positive fungus with short branching mycelia and clusters of blastospores.

It is much more common in females, and presents as whitish or creamy vaginal discharge with vaginal and labial pruritus, redness, excoriations, fissures. Infection may spread to the groins, perineum, and anus. Pregnancy, obesity, diabetes mellitus, malnutrition and prolonged antibiotic or corticosteroid treatment predispose to candidiasis. In males, urethral discharge, redness and soreness of the urethral meatus, and glans penis and pruritus are the main features. Infection may spread to the penile shaft, scrotum, groins and perineum.

Diagnosis

(1) Clinical picture of discharge and local inflammation.
(2) Microscopic examination of smears for *Candida albicans* and other organisms.
(3) Culture of smear in Sabouraud's modified agar medium and isolation of creamy moist colonies of *Candida albicans*.
(4) Serological tests for syphilis, in case both conditions co-exist.

Treatment

Mycostatin vaginal pessaries or vaginal tablets 100,000 units inserted nightly for 2 weeks.
Mycostatin cream externally.
In males, mycostatin cream externally.
Clotrimazole (Canesten) vaginal tablets or cream.

18.8 Virus diseases

Three STD caused by viruses are herpes genitalis, condylomata acuminata (genital warts) and molluscum contagiosum.

Herpes genitalis

This STD is caused by herpes virus hominis, and presents as thin-walled tense vesicles which break within 24–48 hours, leaving small round superficial erosions.

In females, the lesions may be in the cervix, vagina, labia or perineum. They may cause vulval oedema or ulcers or spread in the groins and thighs, causing pain and discomfort. There may be associated fever.

The possible connection of recurrent cervical herpes genitalis with cervical cancer makes this apparently mild STD a potentially dangerous condition.

In males, the vesicles and ulcers appear on the glans penis or prepuce or penile shaft. It is more common in uncircumcised males.

Diagnosis
(1) Clinical picture of vesicles and erosions or herpetic ulcers.
(2) Microscopy and culture of smears for co-existent bacteria.
(3) Isolation of virus, where possible.
(4) Serological tests for syphilis, in case both conditions co-exist.

Treatment There is as yet no specific treatment.
Useful topical applications include:

(1) Antiseptics: silver nitrate solution, potassium permanganate solution, gentian violet, boric acid.
(2) Surgical spirit, ether.
(3) Antibiotics: neomycin, bacitracin, polymyxin, chloramphenicol, oxytetracycline.
(4) Idoxuridine 0.5–40 per cent ointment alone or in combination with dimethylsulphoxide.

Systemic treatment Because of the potential danger of this condition, and the fact that after the superficial lesions have healed, the virus survives in nerve cells and nerve ganglia, some non-specific chemotherapeutic agents have been tried and found useful. These include metronidzole (Flagyl), co-trimoxazole and griseofulvin.

Scrupulous hygiene and the use of antipyretics may cut down on recurrence of herpes genitalis.

Condylomata acuminata *(genital warts)*

This STD is caused by a papilloma virus and presents as dry soft pigmented verrucose plaques on dry surfaces or as moist soft bunched, clustered or fungating masses on mucous surfaces or on muco-cutaneous junctions.

In females, condylomata acuminata may extend into the vagina or cervix. They may become secondarily infected and produce offensive secretions.

Diagnosis
   (1) Clinical picture of verrucose plaques or bunches or clusters or fungating masses.
   (2) Isolation of virus, where possible.
   (3) Biopsy and histopathology.
   (4) Serological tests for syphilis, in case both conditions co-exist.

Treatment
   (1) Podophyllin 10–25 per cent in spirit can be applied to the warts. This is a locally acting cytotoxic drug. The normal skin should be protected while the application is made at night for a number of days until the warts are removed.
   (2) 5-Fluorouracil ointment, another cytotoxic drug. This should also be applied with care.
   (3) Idoxuridine – an anti-viral topical application.
   (4) Chemical destruction with trichloracetic acid, silver nitrate solution or liquor arsenicalis (Fowler's solution).
   (5) Physical removal by curettage, diathermy or excision.

Molluscum contagiosum

This STD is the least common of the three viral infections. It is caused by the molluscum virus and presents as soft glistening globular, dome-shaped or umbilicated papules on the external genitalia, pubic region, perineum, or thighs.
   The papules may become secondarily infected.

Diagnosis
   (1) Clinical picture of characteristic domed or umbilicated papules.
   (2) Isolation of virus, where possible.
   (3) Biopsy and histopathology.
   (4) Serological tests for syphilis, in case both conditions co-exist.

Treatment
   (1) Curettage, touching the bleeding points with liquid phenol, tincture of iodine or tincture of benzoin.
   (2) Diathermy.

18.9   Parasitic infestations

The higher prevalence of scabies and pediculosis pubis among promiscuous or permissive men and women have earned STD ranking for these two parasitic infestations.

18.10   **Venereophobia**

This is a troublesome symptom of fixation in which a patient who may or may not have previously suffered from STD believes that he has STD and wanders from doctor to doctor endlessly seeking treatment for STD.

18.11   **Trends in STD**

Trends in incidence of sexually transmitted diseases vary from one country to another, but on the average, there is currently an upward swing in spite of the availability of effective chemotherapeutic agents and antibiotics.

The permissive society, promiscuity, homosexuality, sex perversion, the use of contraceptive pills and the emergence of resistant mutants of causal organisms are among the factors which hinder the winning of the battle against STD.

Prevention of STD

Vaccination is not successful yet, and popular prophylactic measures such as the wearing of condoms by males, the application of antiseptic creams by females, washing absolutions after sexual intercourse and the swallowing of antibiotics before, during or just after intercourse are all inferior to probity in sex life.

The future of STD

Unless vaccination against STD is achieved, STD will probably remain with man for all time. The merry-go-round will continue, drugs trying to catch up with causal organisms while old and new organisms try to catch up with man's lust for sex with or without love.

19 Principles of Treatment

Most common skin diseases call for direct treatment: the topical application of various preparations – lotions, paints, powders, creams, emulsions, ointments, pastes, sprays. Many require internal medication – antihistamines, antibiotics, tranquilisers, steroids. Some need physical therapy – hydrotherapy, sunlight, ultraviolet rays, various types of X rays. For some skin conditions, surgery is often the best method of treatment – curette, diathermy, excision, cryosurgery.

19.1 Topical treatment

Successful treatment of most common skin diseases can be achieved by intelligent use of a small number of effective topical applications. These applications should be simple in composition, should avoid components likely to sensitise the skin, should be easy to use, and should be as cheap as is compatible with efficacy.

Topical applications are usually made up of biochemically inert bases (vehicles) and active ingredients which the bases transport to the site of their required action. The bases may also be used alone for their physiological action in protecting, lubricating, moistening, drying, cooling or cleansing the skin.

19.2 Bases in common use with or without active ingredients

Ointments These are soft, and spread easily on the skin. They lubricate and soften dry skin, remove debris, and protect the skin against irritation, for example, petrolatum in which various medicaments can be incorporated. The viscosity of ointments can be modified to produce creams, emulsions or pastes.

Creams These are made by decreasing the viscosity of ointments, for example, zinc cream.

Emulsions These are made by adding emulsifying agents to ointments, for example, benzyl benzoate emulsion.

Pastes These are made by adding powders to ointments. Pastes dry as well as protect the skin, for example, Lassar's paste.

Lotions These are made by dissolving or suspending solid substances in water. Lotions cool the skin and, as the water evaporates, the incorporated ingredient is left on the skin, for example, calamine lotion.

Paints These are made by dissolving certain substances in organic solvents such as alcohol or acetone. Paints cool and dry the skin, for example, gentian violet (magenta paint), brilliant green.

Wet dressings The main base is water in which active medicaments are dissolved. Wet dressings dry and cleanse. They may be used as compresses, soaks or baths, for example, potassium permanganate.

Powders These are finely ground substances used for absorbing moisture from and drying the skin, for example, talcum powder.

Shampoos These incorporate medicaments for washing of greasy scalp and other hairy areas, for example, methylated spirit.

Aerosol sprays These are used to deliver incorporated active ingredients under pressure, for example, corticosteroid spray, antibiotic spray.

19.3   Topical medications incorporated in bases

These are usually directed against infections (bacterial, viral, fungal), infestations by animal parasites, and inflammatory, degenerative, auto-immune, neoplastic or other disorders of the skin.

Antibacterial agents For example, antiseptics, astringents, antibiotics. Neomycin, bacitracin and polymyxin which are not commonly given systemically are used singly or in combination as creams, lotions, ointments or sprays.

Antiviral agents For example, idoxuridine, podophyllin.

Antifungal agents For example, Mycostatin (nystatin), clotrimazole.

Antiparasitic agents For example, benzyl benzoate, dicophane (DDT).

Anti-inflammatory agents For example, tar preparations, useful for psoriasis and chronic eczema or dermatitis. Ichthyol is less messy than other tar preparations. Fluorinated and non-fluorinated corticosteroids, are effective in the management of eczema or dermatitis, and many other inflammatory dermatoses. They are easy to use, cosmetically acceptable, do not irritate or sensitise but are still expensive.

Antihistamine preparations For example, mepyramine maleate (Anthisan) promethazine hydrochloride (Phenergan).

Keratolytic agents These help to break down thickened horny layer of the epidermis, for example, salicylic acid.

Caustic agents These are used for the chemical destruction of warts, for example, phenol.

Antimitotic agents These are used for the chemical destruction of tumours in the early stages, for example, 5-fluorouracil.

Photoactive agents These are applied on the skin which is then exposed to sunlight or ultraviolet rays, for example, coal tar, psoralens.

19.4 Systemic treatment

Oral or parenteral treatment may be given to relieve symptoms, to deal with specific infections, inflammatory, degenerative, auto-immune or other disorders, to allay anxiety or as placebo.

Antihistamines These are given for their antipruritic action and sometimes for their soporific side effects, for example, promethazine hydrochloride (Phenergan), mepyramine maleate (Anthisan), chlorpheniramine maleate (Piriton), and diphenhydramine hydrochloride (Benadryl).

Sedatives When sleep is disturbed or there is frank insomnia, sedatives are essential, for example, phenobarbitone, and sodium amytal and butobarbitone (Soneryl).

Tranquilisers In skin disorders associated with stress, tranquilisers should be given, for example, chlorpromazine (Largactil), diazepam (Valium) and chlordiazepoxide (Librium).

Antibiotics Bacterial infections call for prompt and adequate use of antibiotics determined where possible by antibiotic sensitivity tests.

Sulphonamides Sulphapyridine is useful in treating dermatitis herpetiformis.

Antimalarials Chloroquine is used for the treatment of chronic discoid lupus erythematosus and the lucites.

Antifungal antibiotics Fungal infections for which specific antibiotics have been found should be treated with these, for example, griseofulvin for *Microsporon*, *Trichophyton* and *Epidermophyton* infections; Mycostatin (nystatin) for candidiasis.

Amphotericin–B This is a powerful chemotherapeutic agent effective against deep and systemic fungal infections.

Specific parasiticides Diethylcarbamazine citrate (Banocide) is effective against microfiliariae while sodium suramin (Antrypol) is effective against the adult forms of *Onchocerca volvulus*.

Antimycobacterial drugs The standard drug for the treatment of leprosy remains diaminodiphenyl sulphone (dapsone).

Rifampicin and clofazimine though very expensive, are much more effective, and have brightened the prospects in this otherwise grim therapeutic battle. Rifampicin has also joined the traditional front-line drugs (streptomycin, isonicotinic acid hydroxide (INH), para-amino salicylic acid (PAS)) in the treatment of tuberculosis.

Corticosteroids These are useful in the management of severe dermatoses, for example, generalised exfoliative dermatitis, bullous or generalised lichen planus. They are also life-saving in life-threatening conditions such as toxic erythema multiforme (Stevens–Johnson syndrome), toxic epidermal necrolysis (Lyell's disease), systemic lupus erythematosus and pemphigus. Prednisone, prednisolone, triamcinolone, betamethasone and dexamethasone are the most widely used. Their side effects which should be borne in mind include peptic ulceration, exacerbation of hypertension and diabetes mellitus, intercurrent infection, thrombophlebitis, osteoporosis, Cushingoid features and euphoria.

Hormones Severe acne vulgaris in women can sometimes be successfully treated with antiandrogen therapy: oestrogens alone or the oestrogen-progestin combinations in oral contraceptive agents.

Immunosuppressive/antimitotic agents Methotrexate and cyclophosphamide are sometimes effective against auto-immune diseases such as systemic lupus erythematosus and pemphigus. Combinations of methotrexate, cyclophosphamide, and vincristine can also be useful against the leukaemias, lymphomas, mycosis fungoides and Kaposi's sarcoma.

19.5 Physical treatment

Ultraviolet rays The sun is the natural source of ultraviolet rays. When the Prophet Elisha asked the Syrian Army Commander Naaman to 'Go and wash in the River Jordan seven times, and your flesh shall be restored, and you shall be clean', he was pre-empting the current Goeckerman regimen for the treatment of psoriasis with tar baths and ultraviolet light. Tar is a photosensitiser which enhances the action of ultraviolet rays on the erratic keratinisation process in psoriasis. Psoralens given orally also have this photosensitising effect.

X rays Superficial (soft) X rays which interfere with DNA and RNA synthesis and cell replication are used for the treatment of basal-cell carcinoma, squamous-cell carcinoma, and Kaposi's sarcoma.

The much softer Grenz rays can also be used for treating psoriasis and chronic lichenification.

Total body radiation This is a special expensive procedure available only in few special centres for the treatment of mycosis fungoides.

19.6 Surgical treatment

Some skin conditions can be best treated by surgery, usually minor, in a simple theatre attached to the skin clinic.

Excision Under local anaesthesia, skin tags, filarial and other nodules, sebaceous and other cysts, fibromata, lipomata, naevi, warts, keratoses, basal-cell carcinoma, squamous-cell carcinoma, granuloma annulare and other granulomata can be excised.

Major surgical excisions under general anaesthesia may be done for Buruli ulcer, lymphangioma, elephantiasis, and invasive squamous-cell cancer. For malignant melanoma, wide excision with block dissection of lymph nodes is called for. Skin grafting is required when wide areas of skin are excised.

Punch biopsy This modern method of excision uses the biopsy punch for complete removal of small skin lesions 1–5 mm in diameter.

Caustic surgery and cold surgery Warts and molluscum contagiosum can be removed by application of phenol, formalin, podophyllin or other caustic agents. Carbon dioxide snow or liquid nitrogen can also be applied to produce a blister and remove the wart.

Curetting The skin curette can be used to remove warts, molluscum contagiosum, keratoses and small tumours. The bleeding base is thereafter treated with phenol, tincture of iodine or compound tincture of benzoin compound.

Desiccation High frequency diathermy or cutting needles are used to destroy warts or small tumours. The bleeding is taken care of simultaneously and a protective eschar covers the wound.

20 Who Treats Common Skin Diseases?

The eradication or control of the 5-star skin diseases which remain among the scourges of mankind call for crusades mounted by national governments and international organisations.

With dermatologists so few and skin diseases so rampant, doctors should be in the vanguard of programmes to mobilise and train or retrain auxiliary staff from among a wide range of health personnel to help out with routine evaluation and treatment, and with preventive, promotive and educative assignments. This will enable dermatologists to enrich their clinical endeavours with teaching and research, and extend the frontiers of dermatological knowledge.

20.1 National and international crusades

Bacterial infections, fungal infections and infestations by animal parasites which constitute the bulk of skin diseases in many tropical and sub-tropical countries can be fairly considered diseases of underdevelopment and adverse environmental factors. Improvement in socio-economic conditions and education, and control of environmental factors will do much to minimise, control or eradicate some of these diseases and thereby further raise the level of health and improve the quality of life among the people.

Crusades such as have been successfully mounted by the WHO to eradicate the scourges of yaws and smallpox are needed for eradication of other sources such as leprosy and onchocerciasis with blindness (river blindness).

National governments and regional groupings of the affected countries should be in the vanguard of these crusades with the WHO and other international organisations giving their assured support.

20.2 Auxiliary personnel

In many developing countries the doctor to population ratio still ranges from 1:20,000 to 1:100,000. The dermatologist to population ratio may be anything from 1:many millions to nil:the whole population.

Skin diseases comprise 15–20 per cent of diseases presenting in hospitals which are usually situated in or near the urban areas. But about 80–90 per cent of the population in these countries live in the rural areas where poverty is more intense, the standards of domiciliary and environmental hygiene are much lower, and the incidence of skin diseases is expected to be higher.

Given these facts and figures, the questions must arise. Should a dermatologist be treating all patients with skin diseases? Can he afford to? Should all patients with skin diseases be treated by a dermatologist? Can they be so treated? It is true that not only the 5-star skin diseases need expertise. Even trivial and uncomplicated skin diseases need correct diagnosis for correct treatment and, therefore, theoretically need a dermatologist. But expertise for dealing with trivial and uncomplicated skin diseases can safely be taught to non-dermatologists, and the health care of such patients safely delegated to the non-dermatologists.

There is a world-wide shortage of health care professionals. This shortage is much worse in the developing countries where health care has to compete unfavourably with other projects for scarce funds.

The retraining of general practitioners and the training of paramedical personnel to substitute for dermatologists in the care of patients with simple skin diseases, especially in the rural areas, should go some way in solving the problem.

Mobilised and retrained general practitioners, community health physicians and medical officers can be used as supporting teaching staff to help the few dermatologists mount and execute crash training **progra**mmes for nurses and midwives, health visitors and district nurses, school nurses and industrial nurses, health auxiliaries and dispensary assistants, health superintendents and health inspectors, leprosy inspectors and leprosy attendants. The cost of training or retraining of each auxiliary staff should be only a fraction of the cost of training a dermatologist.

Surveys have shown that well trained health auxiliaries working side by side with doctors increase the doctors' productivity. In the face of mounting health problems and population explosion, doctors should not be opposed to delegating responsibilities which can be safely delegated to health personnel with less sophisticated medical training.

Auxiliary health personnel provide primary health care and can be taught to evaluate and solve health problems, and carry out routine curative, preventive, promotive and educative assignments. The role of the doctor remains that of leader and manager of the health team and programme. As his health team increases his effectiveness, he is free to teach and conduct research, and to help mobilise community effort to combat ill health and improve the quality of life in the community.

20.3 **Perspectives**

Dermatology in the tropics can get out of the doldrums of dogmatic statements, myths, misrepresentations and futility only when we have been able to reduce morbidity and been able to find cures or relief for prevalent diseases so that the life of most inhabitants of the tropics can be improved.

In the face of the unequal struggle for scarce funds between health projects on one side and ephemeral prestigious or military program-mes on the other, only enlightened, modest and judicious use of available or readily trainable health personnel can hope to solve a problem which can easily get worse.

Dermatologists in the tropics can get out of the shackling effect of overwhelming numbers of patients only when we are prepared to consider and encourage the rapid development of effective teams of motivated and dedicated auxiliaries. Otherwise, even the more pressing challenges of tropical dermatology such as onchocerciasis with the social and economic consequences of river blindness, leprosy with its psycho-social stigmata and economic handicaps, superficial, deep and systemic fungal infections, viral infections, auto-immune diseases, the lucites, disorders of pigmentation, nutritional disorders, skin tumours and the mounting incidence of eczema or dermatitis cannot be faced squarely. Otherwise, frontier topics in dermatology to which dermatologists in other parts of the world are increasingly turning their attention will all pass us by. These include the immunological aspects of dermatology, metabolic disorders, virus studies, genetic studies, cutaneous ageing, the reticuloses, skin markers of internal diseases and of malignancy, tissue culture, histochemistry and embryology.

In conclusion, the spread of education in dermatology should start with the realisation by the few dermatologists around that we have nothing to lose but our chains if we blaze a trail by championing and organising the widespread and effective training or retraining of auxiliaries from among a wide range of health personnel to help us reduce the load of work in routine mundane dermatology. We have nothing to gain but continuing futility if we continue to keep as a closed shop the drudgery of wallowing in the mud of the dermatology of underdevelopment, and continue to miss the swinging thrill of frontier dermatology and dermatological research and development.

Guides to Further Reading

Borrie, P. F. (ed.) (1975), *Common Skin Diseases*, by A. C. Roxburgh, 14th edition (H. K. Lewis and Co. Ltd, London)

Catterall, R. D. (1979), *Venereology and Genito-urinary medicine* (Hodder and Stoughton, London)

Clarke, G. H. V. (1959), *Skin Diseases in the African* (H. K. Lewis and Co. Ltd, London)

Glickman, Franklin S. (1979), *Dermatology in General Medicine* (P. S. G. Publishing Company Inc., Littleton, Massachusetts)

Hare, P. J. (1966), *Basic Dermatology* (H. K. Lewis and Co. Ltd, London)

King, Ambrose and Nicol, Claude (1975), *Venereal Diseases* (Bailliere Tindall, London)

Levene, G. M. and Calnan, C. D. (1974), *A Colour Atlas of Dermatology* (Wolfe Medical Books, London)

Marshall, James (1960), *Diseases of the Skin* (E. and S. Livingstone Ltd, Edinburgh and London)

Rook, A., Wilkinson, D. S., and Ebling, F. J. G. (1972), *Textbook of Dermatology* (Blackwell Scientific Publications, Oxford)

Sauer, Gordon C. (1973), *Manual of Skin Diseases* (J. B. Lippincott Company, Philadelphia and Toronto)

Sneddon, I. B. and Church, R. E. (1976), *Practical Dermatology* (Edward Arnold, London)

Stewart, Wm. D., Danto, Julius L., and Maddin Stuart (1978), *Dermatology*, 4th edition (C. V. Mosby Company, St. Louis)

Index